Practicing Buddhism in Everyday Life

Nicole Dake

Dedication

I would like to dedicate this book to my family and my best friends, who are like family. This is for Atlantis, River, Gary, Aubrey, and Debbie, who listen to my spiritual musings and accept them without question. Thank you for all your support of my writing journey and my spiritual journey as well.

I hope that my practice of Buddhism in my life helps me be a calmer and more whole person who is able to give back to you in all the beautiful ways that you have given to me over the years.

I love you all, and I couldn't do this without your love and support.

Acknowledgment

This book couldn't have been written without the wonderful coaching support that I received from Tanvi Chadha. Thank you for the mindset coaching that you did with me; it helped me to get back into Buddhism and practice Mindfulness and Meditation on a daily basis. This has been the foundation not only for this book but for getting my life back on track when I was floundering.

I would also like to thank my wonderful Beta Readers, Art Bram, and Michele Maize. I really appreciate your support with this book and the wonderful feedback that you provided me with. It is so wonderful to have support from within the writing community. I am lucky and blessed to have gotten to know both of you. Thank you again for taking the time to help me with this project.

Contents

Dedication iii

Acknowledgment iv

Preface.. viii

Introduction: How Mindset Coaching Helped Me Become More
Mindful and Find Inner Peace...............................1

　　Taking a Leap of Faith 3

　　The Course Content 5

　　Impact on My Life 7

　　My Partner's Perspective............................. 10

　　Conclusion 13

Foundations of Buddhism 15

　　Four Noble Truths Explained................................. 17

These Buddhist Practices Have Been Validated by Science30

Practicing Mindfulness Can Help Ease Stress 36

What is Mindfulness? 38

　　Mindful Presence 39

Benefits of Mindfulness..................................48

　　Mindfulness increases happiness 52

　　Mindfulness helps us to fully experience life 53

　　Mindfulness helps with Anxiety and Depression 54

　　Mindfulness helps us be better parents.................. 55

　　Mindfulness makes us more productive 56

　　Mindfulness improves our relationships............................. 57

Practicing Mindfulness 59

Beginners Mind is Key to a Growth Mindset 63

Mindful Parenting: How To Be Present In The Moment With Your Child...67

    Put Away Your Phone 67

    Transformational Listening.. 70

    Mindful Parenting 72

    Conclusion 74

Mindfulness Quotes to Help You Become a More Peaceful, Happy, and Loving Parent 75

Mindfulness Quotes 77

Conclusion 81

Yoga..83

My Favorite Way to Relieve Stress Is Doing Yoga...........83

Health Benefits of Yoga..85

    Emotional Benefits of Yoga 86

    Spiritual Benefits of Yoga 89

Getting Started With Yoga...94

Different styles of Yoga...96

    Conclusion 102

Practicing Yoga..103

Meditation...106

Meditation can help ease stress and calm your mind.......106

Other Benefits of Meditation 112

How to Meditate 114

Chant the "Om" and Remember how to Fly....................118

The Search to Reclaim Inner Peace 123

Closing Thoughts 126

References...128

About the Author 131

Preface

Buddhism is more than a religion; it is a way of life. As a practice-based religion, it is easy to incorporate Buddhism into your everyday life without having to attend religious services, classes, or read through a bunch of theology. (Although you definitely can if that interests you!) In this book, I will only briefly discuss the core ideas of Buddhism so that you will have a grasp of the concepts before I delve straight into the practice section.

This book is focused on Mindfulness, Meditation, and Yoga, which are core Buddhist practices that can greatly improve your life. All of these practices have benefits to your life that are validated by scientific research as well.

Modern Buddhism is very East-Meets-West because of the convergence of religion and science when it comes to the day-to-day practices that Buddhists use to improve their mindset and their life.

The end goal of Buddhism is to achieve spiritual enlightenment, ease your suffering, and break out of the cycle of death and rebirth. But even if you don't achieve your mountain-top moment in this lifetime, there are still huge daily benefits to practicing Buddhism that we will discuss throughout this book.

You don't need to go anywhere or buy anything to get started. All you need to do is prepare to go within yourself and deepen your understanding of yourself, the world, and how you relate to the world with a sense of peace. This is a journey of self-exploration. I hope that you will enjoy these Buddhist practices as much as I do and that they will greatly enhance your life.

Introduction:
How Mindset Coaching Helped Me Become
More Mindful and Find Inner Peace

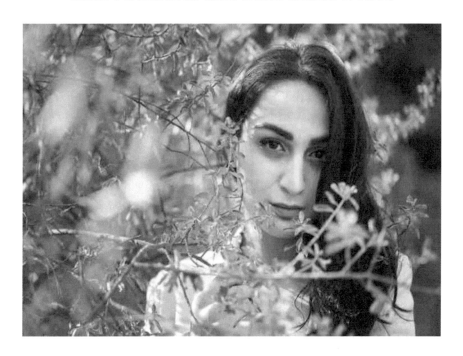

Tanvi, the coach at We Wear Wellness

It was a mindset coaching program that led me back to Buddhism, back to Mindfulness and Meditation, and back to myself.

Sometimes in life, we are looking for something without really realizing what it is. I was looking for answers to why my life felt so empty. I had everything that I was 'supposed' to have in life. The whole dream of the white picket fence life in the suburbs. Only it felt like something was missing. Everything was 'fine', but I was tired of fine. I wanted more.

Only, I came to realize that more, in this case, was less. What I really wanted most of all was to simplify and return to listening to my inner voice. It was telling me that all the stuff, all the trappings of life, weren't what I really wanted. I wanted spiritual realization. I wanted inner peace.

More *stuff* will never help you find spiritual realization.

There is an old saying that "when the student is ready, the teacher will appear." I have found that to be true in my own life.

My inner longing was what led me to start a coaching program that would spur me on the path to finding inner peace and spiritual realization. Of all places, I found my coach, Tanvi, on Instagram. Even with the whole influencer culture there, there is a lot of spirituality and positivity on Instagram, too.

About a year ago, I enrolled in the program called Burnout to Badass, with coaching provided by Tanvi Chadha of <u>We Wear Wellness</u>. On her website, she states her mission as, "I help ambitious women who struggle with negativity, overwhelm, and anxiety, to transform their mindset by shifting their limiting beliefs, and embody the BEST version of themselves through the power of SELF-LOVE!"

First, I started following Tanvi's We Wear Wellness account for all the positivity that I found there. She was so happy and upbeat that I was drawn to her energy right away! When she advertised in one of her videos that she had 4 coaching spots open, I emailed her right away because I wanted one of them. I needed to find out how to create an infectious, beautiful energy like that for myself!

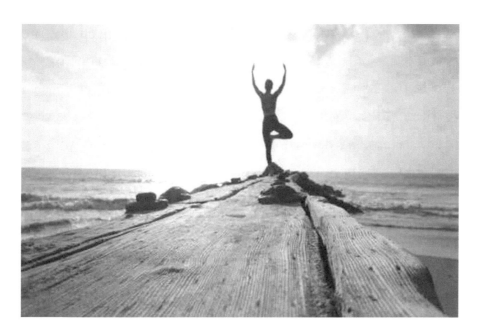

Taking a Leap of Faith

Deciding to radically change your life is like taking a leap of faith. For several months, I had felt like I was standing on the brink of an inner change. Like I was looking at puzzle pieces of the answers to life all laid out before me, and I just had to figure out how to put them together. Signing up for the Burnout to Badass course was my leap of faith.

I asked both my partner and my teen daughter the same question before I decided to sign up. I asked them, "Will you still want to be with me if I make a big change in myself?" I got different and interesting answers from both.

Gary replied back to me and said, "If you make a big change, are you still going to want to be with ME?" I told him yes. I don't know if he was actually reassured, but we have the kind of relationship where we are completely open and honest with each other. The good and the bad. We decided that I had been struggling a lot with my panic attacks and coping with past trauma, and it was bleeding over into our family life. So he told me that a positive change for me would be a positive change for all of us.

Atlantis told me, "Mom, I have been with you through so many changes already. I will be with you no matter what." I love my girl. Sometimes the way she reacts to the big things in life, and takes them in stride, makes me think of her as an old soul.

After talking through things with the family (minus River, I don't know that a 4-year-old would understand a coaching class) I told

Tanvi yes, I was in. I was committed to making a real change in my life, excited and nervous about it.

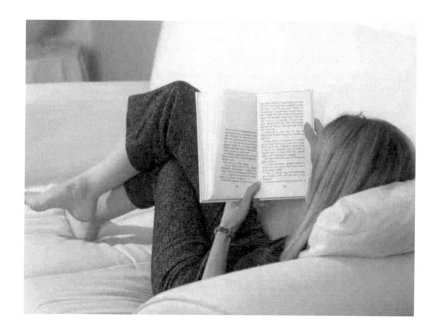

Weekly reading and writing activities.

The Course Content

Every Monday morning (adjusted for the different time zones), Tanvi would email me with a new workbook and video for that week. I would watch the video, think it through overnight, and then start work on the workbook the next day. In addition to the workbook, the video would give one or two skills to work on that week.

In the beginning, it was lowering your to-do list, journaling and self-care. The premise is that if you are feeling overwhelmed, you will need to take things off your plate that are causing you stress.

Many of the interim weeks talked about limiting beliefs, working through your triggers, and a lot of introspection. Everything was interwoven with themes of Mindfulness.

Since I had studied Buddhism before, I was familiar with the concept of Mindful Presence, but I was unfamiliar with the non-judgment aspect of Mindfulness. Connecting with this beautiful, peaceful energy really helped me to come home to myself.

I did a lot of writing, a lot of thinking, and had a lot of long talks with my partner about the changes I needed to make in my inner world.

Changing your life isn't so much about changing the outer world. First, you have to change your inner world and the way that you think about the things that are happening every day. Once you have changed your mindset and your thinking, then you can start changing the outer world.

One of the great things about the class is that every week, in every workbook and video, Tanvi spoke about the scientific research base of the practices that I was learning. Everything that you think, how your mind works, has a basis in neuroscience. As someone who had taken neuropsychology courses in college, it resonated with me.

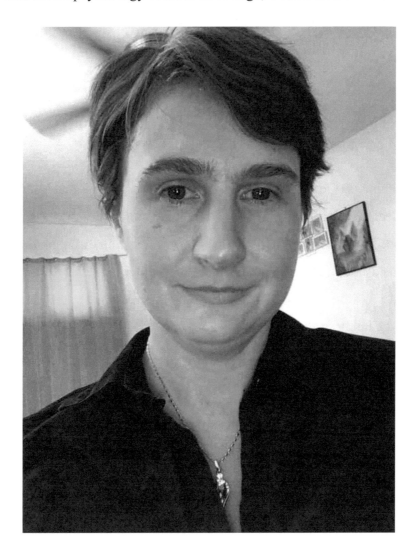

I am so much happier!

Impact on My Life

I bet you guys are all wondering if I was really able to find inner peace in a 12-week class. It sounds impossible, right? I'm not the Buddha sitting under the Bodhi tree, after all.

Well, I didn't need the Bodhi tree; I didn't need the mountain top. I found inner peace by week 4. Honestly, I had experienced it before that, but in glimpses, that would come and go. My goal for the program was to learn to hold onto inner peace.

The thing is, I realized that inner peace isn't something that you can hold onto. I was grasping at something that wasn't meant to be grasped. Inner peace is about letting go—like taking the leap of faith I talked about earlier—and realizing that inner peace is our true nature. We are all part of life's heart. Pure, perfect love. Pure, perfect life. I came to it through acceptance. Accepting my circumstances, accepting my life as it is, and letting go of all the judgments of good or bad that had been holding me back.

I also learned self-love. It was a struggle for me since I spent a big part of my life being a very self-hating person. Again, it comes down to acceptance, gentleness, and that pure, perfect love.

The experience of this kind of love is something that is beyond words. They say, "Those who know do not speak. Those who speak do not know."

However, I will use this book to try to convey that feeling of inner peace, self-love, and self-acceptance that I have found through these Buddhist practices.

The more you allow this pure, perfect love to permeate your life, the more peaceful you will become. You realize that you are a piece of life's heart. A cell within the body of the Universe. And this boundless, loving energy is what you are made of.

Everything is made up of energy, according to science. This is very like the concept of Prana (life force) within Buddhism. Energy is what makes up everything, us included. The more we become aware of and in tune with this energy, the more our lives become an effortless flow.

My relationships improved too. Now that I am not feeling emotionally depleted, I have more to give to my family. I can be more present with my partner and my girls and more able to play. More able to be compassionate to their needs and give them what they need too. Improving yourself improves the way that you relate to others.

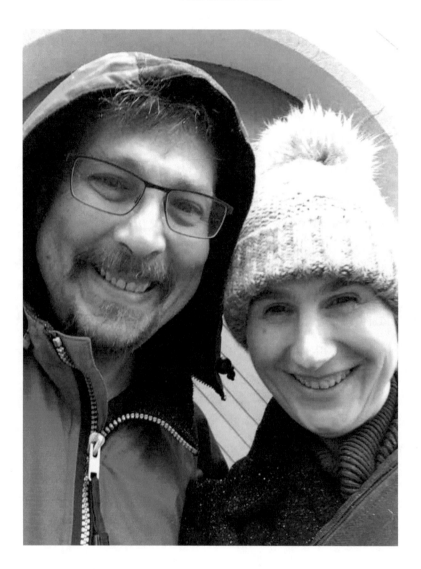

My Partner's Perspective

While I was taking this course, I talked to Gary about what I was learning and the changes I wanted to make in myself. Sometimes our talks were good, sometimes less so when I was struggling with things that I wanted to fix.

We always keep an open door in our relationship to talk about anything and everything. Sometimes the way I talk to him is really a stream of consciousness, the good and the bad.

At the end, though, I asked him if he thought I seemed any different. He said yes, I seem a lot happier and less reactive. He said that he could see that this class really helped me, that I enjoyed it, and that it was money well spent.

NICOLE DAKE

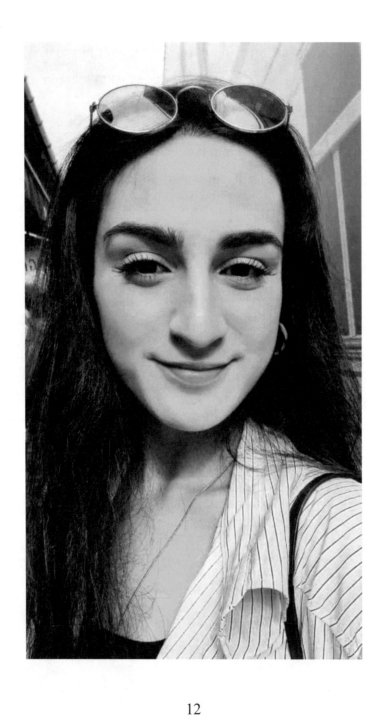

PRACTICING BUDDHISM IN EVERYDAY LIFE

Are you ready to be a badass?

Conclusion

I realized things with Tanvi, because of the way she phrased things to me, that I hadn't realized in years of therapy. To me that is HUGE. It was so helpful how Tanvi used the language of Buddhism and Mindfulness with me since that is something I was already familiar with.

I also achieved some wonderful spiritual realizations. I believe that in Tanvi, I truly have found a <u>Sadguru</u> who has helped me find a deeply spiritual path. I don't know that she would describe herself this way, but truly she has helped me to find the final step on the path to inner peace.

Your goals direct your course. You find the answers that YOU need. The answer that I needed was to look within, find mindfulness, and return to my spirituality.

Throughout this book, I hope that you find a way to connect - or reconnect - with your spirituality as well. You can find spirituality and spiritual experience in everyday life. You don't have to be an extraordinary person or do extraordinary things. All you have to do is find a quiet place to sit in your own house, then spend some time there.

By exploring the themes of Mindfulness, Meditation and Yoga, I hope that you will be able to find some spiritual realizations through your practice the way that I have!

Thank you for reading, my lovelies!

Foundations of Buddhism

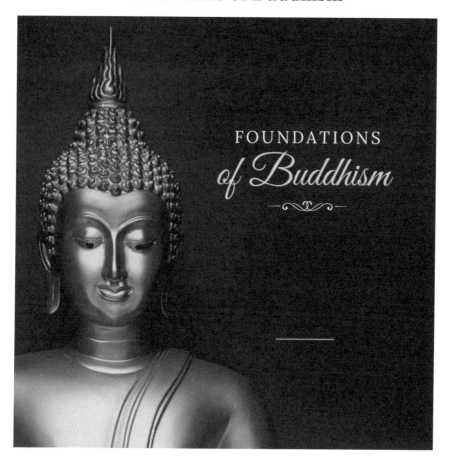

Buddhism is an ancient religion that was founded in India by followers of the Buddha. The focus of this religion is achieving enlightenment and mental peace.

Many of the practices in Buddhism are still applicable to us today and have been validated by science as having a practical value in our lives in addition to their spiritual value.

Before I delve into these practices, meditation, mindfulness and yoga, I am going to share some of the main principles of Buddhism. This way, you will understand the foundational beliefs of this religion so that you are better able to put them into practice.

One of the main tenets of Buddhism is the Four Noble Truths. These are the foundational beliefs within Buddhism.

The four Noble Truths are:

1. The truth of the Suffering *(dukkha sacca)*
2. The truth of the cause of the Suffering *(dukkha-samudāya sacca)*
3. The truth of the cessation the Suffering *(dukkha-nirodha sacca)*
4. The truth of the way leading to the cessation of Suffering *(dukkha-nirodha-gamini-paṭipadā sacca)*

Four Noble Truths Explained

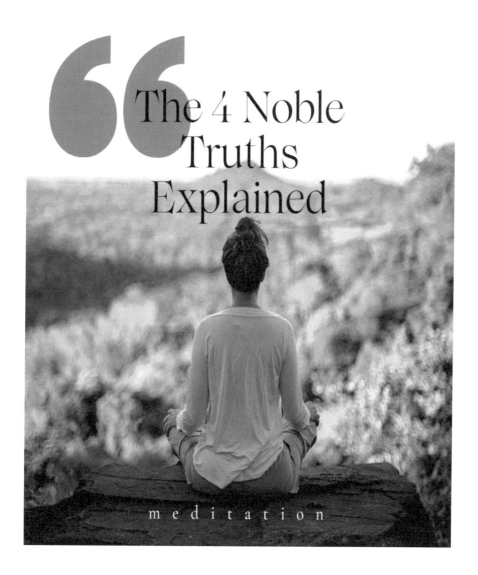

NICOLE DAKE

The First Noble Truth

According to Buddho, the Buddha teaches that,

> *"Now this, bhikkhus, is the noble truth of suffering: birth is suffering, aging is suffering, illness is suffering, death is suffering; union with what is displeasing is suffering; separation from what is pleasing is suffering; not to get what one wants is suffering; in brief, the five aggregates subject to clinging are suffering."*

We can't possibly avoid suffering. It is a part of life, just like breathing. Everyone suffers from old age and death eventually, even if they don't suffer for other reasons before that.

The Buddha was raised as a prince, and when he went out into the city for the first time, he saw an old person, a sick person, and someone who had died. This was the first time that he realized that bad things could happen because he had been so isolated growing up.

Then, he went on to meditate on suffering and try to understand the place that suffering holds in our lives.

The Second Noble Truth

According to <u>Buddho</u>, the Buddha tells us,

> "Now this, bhikkhus, is the noble truth of the origin of suffering: it is this craving which leads to renewed existence, accompanied by delight and lust, seeking delight here and there; that is, craving for sensual pleasures, craving for existence, craving for extermination."

> "And where does this desire come from and take root? Wherever in the world there are pleasurable and enjoyable things, this desire arises and takes root. Eye, ear, nose, tongue, body and consciousness are pleasurable and enjoyable; that is where this desire comes from and takes root."

> "Visual objects, sounds, smells, taste, touch and mental objects are pleasurable and enjoyable; that's where this desire comes from and takes root."

> "Consciousness, sensory impressions, feelings arising from the sensory impressions, perception, intention, craving, thinking and reflecting are pleasurable and enjoyable, that's

where this desire comes in and takes root."

"This is the second noble truth."

When we suffer, it is because we aren't getting what we want. Suffering comes from the opposite of what has been our pleasures in life.

The Buddha tells us that suffering comes from craving. This means when we want something, it causes us to suffer. We want things so badly that we have blinders on to all the goodness that is already around us. We are living in the future instead of the present.

We have gotten attached in our minds to some certain outcome, and if we don't get that desired outcome, then we are upset, and we suffer.

No one can get what they want all the time. That means we are destined to suffer as long as we are allowing ourselves to want things.

The Third Noble Truth

According to <u>Buddho</u>, the Buddha tells us,

> *"Now this, bhikkhus, is the noble truth of the cessation of suffering: it is the remainderless fading away and cessation of that same craving, the giving up and relinquishing of it, freedom from it, non-reliance on it."*

We can stop suffering if we release our cravings and attachments. When we stop being attached to the outcomes of a situation, we are no longer suffering. That is because we have made it, so our internal state isn't attached to circumstances anymore.

The Buddha teaches that we can reach enlightenment when we stop being attached to outcomes.

If we aren't attached to what happens, our feelings aren't dependent on situations anymore. We aren't happy or sad based on what is happening anymore, so we have stopped suffering.

The Fourth Noble Truth

According to <u>Buddho</u>, the Buddha tells us,

> *"Now this, bhikkhus, is the noble truth of the way leading to the cessation of unsatisfactoriness: it is this Noble Eightfold Path; that is, right view (sammā diṭṭhi), right intention (sammā saṅkappa), right speech (sammā vācā), right action (sammā kammanta), right livelihood (sammā ājīva), right effort (sammā vāyāma), right mindfulness (sammā sati) and right concentration (sammā samādhi)."*

By getting into the right mindset using the eightfold path, we can stop our suffering. This is how we find enlightenment. Enlightenment is the way to be free of suffering, according to the teachings of the Buddha.

Some of the ways to follow the eightfold path are through using practices like mindfulness, meditation and yoga.

Even if we don't follow the complete eightfold path, these practices are very useful in learning to become happier in life. These practices help us to be more present at the moment instead of immersed in our cravings, which lead to suffering.

When You Practice Buddhism, it Becomes a Part of You

Buddhism is based on practice instead of on belief.

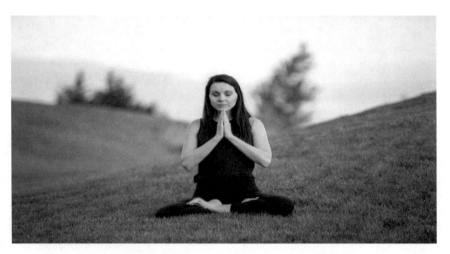

Photo by <u>Benjamin Child</u> on <u>Unsplash</u>

After practicing Buddhism for years, it becomes a part of you. I suppose it is that way with any religion.

Buddhism is based on practices such as <u>meditation</u>, <u>mindfulness</u>, and <u>yoga</u>. In Japanese Buddhism, there are additional mindful practices such as flower arrangement, calligraphy and the tea ceremony.

Practice-Based vs. Faith-Based

When you are a Buddhist, your religion centers around what you do much more than what you believe. When I was a Christian, it was all about belief.

A long time ago, a Buddhist Monk said to me, "Practice your religion, and practice it every day."

Of course, at the time, I was only 16 years old, so I didn't really understand the depth of that statement. It was part of a tour of a Buddhist Temple that my class had gone to for school, and the monk was speaking to a group of primarily secular teenagers.

Yet, over 20 years later, that statement sticks with me.

Firstly, because he wasn't trying to convert us to Buddhism, he was telling us to practice *our* religion, whatever that may have been at the time.

Secondly, it sticks with me because of the very idea of *practice*. The term practice implies that we shouldn't expect perfection. Every day we are simply practicing. We can constantly improve ourselves and our practice. We don't need to pressure ourselves to be perfect; we can allow our practice to flow naturally.

When I was a Christian, everything was about the belief system. You can see this today, even in the news media. Christians are focused on converting other people to their same belief system and worldview.

The focus is on beliefs instead of actions. "For it is by grace you have been saved, through faith—and this is not from yourselves, it is the gift of God—not by works so that no one can boast." **(Ephesians 2:8–9)**.

As a Christian, I went to church several times a week to hear sermons about how I was supposed to live my life. We spent time studying and reading the Bible and singing hymns of praise to God. It was a passive religion instead of an active one.

Buddhism Becomes a Part of You

After a while, Buddhist practices become a part of you.

I was reminded of this as I stood on my porch this morning and saw my Buddha statue in my snow-covered garden.

Every morning, I wake up and start the day with yoga. Every night, I meditate on chants of "Om Mani Padme Hum" before I go to bed. My watch even has a setting for mindful moments that I can practice throughout the day.

> "We are what we repeatedly do. Excellence, then, is not an act but a habit."
>
> — Will Durant

PRACTICING BUDDHISM IN EVERYDAY LIFE

As we form these mindful habits, it allows us to embrace the fullness of ourselves and to enrich our lives through practice. After a while, we don't think so much about the source of our habits; we just flow through them.

That's how it is for me with my morning yoga. I don't think about the purpose of yoga. I don't think about why I started doing yoga. I don't think about the thousands of years of history of the yogis who practiced before me. My mind is like a blank slate, focusing on the breath, flowing through the familiar poses.

When you go to a Buddhist temple, it's quiet. You may walk in to find a giant statue of a Buddha or an altar where people place offerings like prayer scrolls. It is different around the world, but the quiet is the same. People sit in meditation or prayer. Quiet contemplation.

True, sometimes there will be talks or meditation classes. Frequently, these will be quiet too. The instructor sits and guides you through the practice, then invites you to practice daily at home as well.

In the words of one of my favorite yogis, Sarah Beth, "Your daily practice is your strongest practice."

In a Faith-Based Religion, it is Different

When you practice a faith-based religion like Christianity, you are asked to constantly reflect on your beliefs. There is constant reading, study, and sermonizing. Constantly, they are telling you what to believe.

They preach about heaven and hell. About guarding your heart against sin. They use fear to tell you that you have to act a certain way or you are going to hell. One could argue that this is a practice as well, the constant focus on not sinning.

There is Christianity in theory, which is often different from Christianity in practice. Many people who call themselves Christians haven't been to church in years, but they still *believe*.

For them, it is the belief that is important. " If you declare with your mouth, "Jesus is Lord," and believe in your heart that God raised him from the dead, you will be saved. For it is with your heart that you believe and are justified, and it is with your mouth that you profess your faith and are saved." (**Romans 10:9–10**)

This is one of the central tenets of Christianity, and it mentions nothing about how one should act in daily life.

PRACTICING BUDDHISM IN EVERYDAY LIFE

There are many comparisons throughout the years of the Buddha and Christ. One major example of this is the book <u>Living Buddha, Living Christ</u>. It compares the actions and sermons of the two while they were alive, and they were actually quite similar.

It is interesting to see how two figures who focused on teaching love and compassion in their lifetimes have become the leading figures in such ideologically different religions.

These Buddhist Practices Have Been Validated by Science

Do you want to improve your mindset and your life? These ancient practices can help.

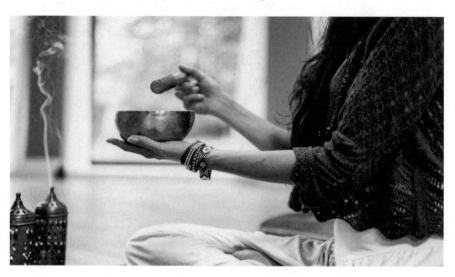

Photo by <u>Conscious Design</u> on <u>Unsplash</u>

In this increasingly busy and technologically connected world, it is important to unplug and connect with your body and mind.

The ancient Buddhist practices of Mindfulness, Yoga and Meditation can help you go within and find balance in your mind and body.

In recent years, scientific studies have validated the usefulness of these Buddhist meditative practices to combat stress, anxiety and depression. Now, they are also recommended by many psychologists for your mental health and wellness.

Meditation

Practicing meditation is one of the easiest things that you can do to decrease stress and improve your mental health.

You don't need any equipment, just a quiet place to sit. Then, you place your hands on your knees, close your eyes, and focus on your breathing.

Sounds easy, right?

According to the National Center for <u>Complimentary and Integrative Health</u>,

> Meditation and mindfulness practices may have a variety of health benefits and may help people improve the quality of their lives. Recent studies have investigated if meditation or mindfulness helps people manage anxiety, stress, depression, pain, or symptoms related to withdrawal from nicotine, alcohol, or opioids.

> Other studies have looked at the effects of meditation or mindfulness on weight control or sleep quality.

31

With all these proven benefits, meditation can be great not just for your mental health but your physical health as well. It can be great to start a meditation practice right away!

According to The Harvard Gazette,

> Desbordes' research uses functional magnetic resonance imaging (fMRI), which not only takes pictures of the brain, as a regular MRI does but also records brain activity occurring during the scan. In 2012, she demonstrated that changes in brain activity in subjects who have learned to meditate hold steady even when they're not meditating. Desbordes took before-and-after scans of subjects who learned to meditate over the course of two months. She scanned them not while they were meditating but while they were performing everyday tasks. The scans still detected changes in the subjects' brain activation patterns from the beginning to the end of the study, the first time such a change—in a part of the brain called the amygdala—had been detected.

This is important research because it shows that a meditation practice can benefit you in your day-to-day activities, as well as when you are meditating!

PRACTICING BUDDHISM IN EVERYDAY LIFE

Mindfulness

Mindfulness is the practice of being fully aware of the present moment. You observe all that is around you and immerse yourself in being present without judging your thoughts.

You can choose to be mindful at any time, in any place. All you have to do is focus on your body, your breath, and your environment. You can be mindfully present during any activity that you are participating in.

According to the American Psychological Association,

> Many studies show that practicing mindfulness reduces stress. In 2010, Hoffman et al. conducted a meta-analysis of 39 studies that explored the use of mindfulness-based stress reduction and mindfulness-based cognitive therapy. The researchers concluded that mindfulness-based therapy may be useful in altering affective and cognitive processes that underlie multiple clinical issues.

> Those findings are consistent with evidence that mindfulness meditation increases positive affect and decreases anxiety and negative affect.

So, according to this study, you can see that the results show that you will have more 'positive affect,' which means that you will be happier. This is a great benefit to such a simple practice!

Yoga

Practicing yoga is a bit more difficult than Meditation or Mindfulness because it is like a meditation that is tied to physical poses.

When you practice yoga, you go through a series of poses, connecting your body to your breathing. It is like a combination of Meditation and exercise, connecting your body and mind through a focus on your breathing.

According to Medical News Today,

> According to scientific research, yoga may:
>
> - reduce stress
> - relieve anxiety
> - help manage depression
> - decrease lower back pain
> - improve quality of life in those with chronic conditions or acute illnesses
> - stimulate brain function
> - help prevent heart disease

When trying yoga for the first time, join a class for beginners under the direction of a qualified instructor to avoid injuries.

These are wonderful physical and mental health benefits that you can experience as you try a yoga practice for yourself.

After learning about all the physical and mental health benefits of the ancient Buddhist practices of Meditation, Mindfulness and Yoga, it seems like the monks may be onto something!

I use all these practices in my daily life and experience huge benefits from all of them. I would highly recommend trying them yourself.

NICOLE DAKE

Mindfulness

Practicing Mindfulness Can Help Ease Stress

The Buddhist practice of mindfulness has many scientific benefits for stress reduction

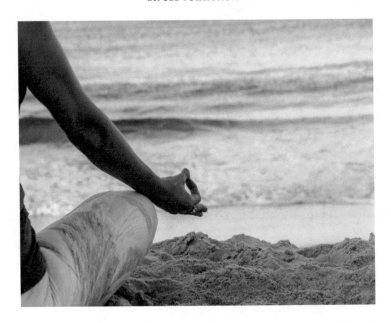

Photo by Chelsea Gates on Unsplash

Mindfulness has many benefits to our daily lives in this stressful and fast-paced modern world.

Being mindful can help us be more present and connected to the present moment instead of dwelling on our stressful and anxious thoughts. We can allow our thoughts to flow without judgment

36

and release them.

These are the basics of mindfulness practice. You can do this for only minutes a day and gradually expand mindfulness to more areas of your life.

What is Mindfulness?

<u>Mindfulness</u> has two aspects to it: being present and non-judgment. When we are fully present at the moment, we see things exactly as they are. We don't think of them as being good or bad; we see the beauty in everything. Mindfulness is seeing everything with new eyes, like a child, for the first time.

When we allow ourselves to be mindfully present, we can experience the world more fully. It helps us to be better parents because we are fully present with our children, without our thoughts wandering off. We pay more attention to them and cultivate our parenting relationship more fully.

When we are more present in each moment of the day, it suddenly feels like we do have more time because we aren't constantly distracted.

So, in moments when you want to be more mindful, you can focus on one of these mindfulness quotes. Then, focus on being completely present with what you are doing right now.

Don't think about the past or worry about the future. Just be fully present right where you are, with what you are doing.

Taking these mindful moments throughout the day helps you to center and refocus your energy. Back to yourself. Back to your kids. Back to the task at hand.

I have found when I apply this principle in my daily life, it helps me to be more mindful and at peace in my daily life.

Mindful Presence

Learning to practice mindfulness with life itself, and with our parenting in particular, can counteract our busy culture of being on the phone all the time.

The basics of mindfulness are outlined in <u>Mindful Adventure,</u>

> *[there are] seven specific attitudes that form a foundation for mindfulness. They apply directly, moment by moment and day by day, as you cultivate and deepen mindfulness. These attitudes are **non-judging, patience, beginner's mind, trust, non-striving, acceptance** and **letting go.** The attitudes support each other and are deeply interconnected. Practicing one will lead to the others. Your ability to bring*

these attitudes forward in your mindfulness practice will have a great deal to do with your long-term success and ability to calm your anxious mind.

The first part of Mindfulness is the idea of Beginners Mind, which can also be referred to as being mindfully present. It is being in the moment and paying attention only to what is going on around you without worrying about the future or the past.

According to <u>Mindful Adventure,</u>

When you begin to observe what is here in the present moment, the thinking mind tends to believe it knows all about what is happening, or it tries to control what is happening by desperately seeking more information. The activity of thinking forms a kind of filter between you and the direct experience and true richness of life as it unfolds moment by moment.

To practice a beginner's mind means to be open to the experience in each moment as if meeting it for the first time. Imagine the wonder of a child as she encounters something for the first time. The first smell of a flower, the first drop of rain, the first taste of an orange; are all experienced without the intermediate layer of thought or comparison to the past. These moments are experienced just as they are, in the now, directly, as smell or touch or taste, as sound or sight. In truth, each moment is unique.

To practice Beginner's Mind is to see the world as a child sees it. How much better to connect with them when you can look at the world with wonder as they do instead of thinking in the back of your mind about your to-do list!

What is Beginner's Mind?

The beginner's mind is a Buddhist concept that is used in the practice of Mindfulness.

When you practice mindfulness, you look at the world around you while being fully present and not judging your thoughts or experiences.

According to Zen Habits,

> What is a beginner's mind? It's dropping our expectations and preconceived ideas about something and seeing things with an open mind and fresh eyes, just like a beginner. If you've ever learned something new, you can remember what that's like you're probably confused because you don't know how to do whatever you're learning, but you're also looking at everything as if it's brand new, perhaps with curiosity and wonder.

41

That's a beginner's mind.

The beginner's mind is seeing everything as an alien or as a child, as if for the first time. It is taking time to truly see and appreciate everything around you. Look at things as if you have never seen them before, with curiosity and openness.

A return to beginner's mind was an exercise that Tanvi had me do in the Burnout to Badass program, and it really helped me to reconnect with the world around me.

As you practice beginner's mind, your attributions and judgments about why things are the way they are beginning to melt away. You can look at the world around you without all of your preconceived ideas about the reasons behind things.

Non-Judgement

The second aspect of mindfulness, which I alluded to briefly in the introduction of this chapter, is non-judgment.

Typically, as we spend our day thinking various thoughts, we are also judging our thoughts as being good or bad. Oftentimes, it is our judgments about our thoughts that upset us, not the actual thoughts of ourselves.

We have a tendency to attach to the thoughts that we perceive as good, resist the thoughts that we perceive as bad, and ignore the thoughts that are neutral. This means we are treating each thought in a different way based on our judgment of that thought. This can lead us to follow some thoughts much more closely than others.

With positive thoughts, we get a dopamine high from them, so we chase them in search of more.

Since we ignore the neutral thoughts and let them float away unattended to, this means that we are ignoring a large portion of our thoughts and judging them to be unimportant. This can be problematic because neutral thoughts would allow us to live a more peaceful existence if we would pay more attention to them.

We can also attach to negative thoughts in the form of a negative judgment spiral in our minds.

For example, if I was thinking about how I need to clean up my kitchen but that I don't really want to clean up the kitchen, I might judge the second part as a bad thought. I then would get into a spiral of self-judgment about how I am a bad person because I don't want to clean up my kitchen.

This spiral of judgments leads to a lot of negative self-talk, which could easily be avoided if I hadn't:

1. Judged my thoughts as good or bad
2. Spiraled out of control by judging myself based on my thoughts

Throughout our day, there are hundreds of thoughts that flow through our minds. If we judge each of these and spiral out of control every time we have a thought we judge to be bad, then we are heaping a lot of unnecessary criticism onto ourselves all day long.

So much negative thinking and negative self-talk can lead to quite a lot of suffering in our lives. All because of simply thinking and allowing ourselves to attach judgments to our thoughts. Then we pile on additional judgments to the judgments. It is a wonder, with thinking like this, that we get anything done during the day at all!

When we learn to practice non-judgment, we suspend the judgment of our thoughts as good or bad. We allow them simply to be.

According to Mindful Ambition,

> *The last part of that definition, non-judgment, means **letting***

go of the automatic judgments that arise in your mind with every experience you have.

Setting down the judging mind, even for a short while, is a refreshing weight off of your shoulders.

In practicing non-judgment, there's no longer anything to be done about the present moment. No grasping for more, no resisting what's there, and no ignoring life's experience.

When you stop trying to react to your experience, you can open up to it completely, resting in mindful presence.

When we practice non-judgment, it allows our minds to rest and to be at peace. We can just let our thoughts flow past without attaching to them in some specific way. This allows us to be more Mindfully Present as well.

Mindful Ambition also lists some benefits of non-judgment:

- **Non-judgment opens you up to more of life's beauty.** Judging something as "neutral" means it's not worth your attention. But when you remove this judgment of "neutral", you have the chance to see the beauty and wonder present in every aspect of life. Any activity can be a wonderful, enriching experience if you take the time to pay attention to it.

- **Non-judgment helps you off the hedonic treadmill**. So much dissatisfaction comes from the endless quest for *more*. Be it money, accomplishments, or titles, the motivation of that pursuit comes from the judgment that what you have now is not enough. Letting go of that judgment, you can appreciate the countless positive qualities of where you are now.

- **Non-judgment helps you cultivate a peaceful mind.** Your judgments are the only source of stress about the "bad" things in your life, or whatever might happen in the future. Letting go of the judgment of "bad" frees you from the suffering caused by interpreting it this way.

- **Non-judgment helps you see clearly.** When reacting to your judgments, you're only seeing your interpretation of what's there. Letting go of those judgments helps you see things as they actually are.

The more we can learn to practice non-judgment of our thoughts as a part of our daily experience, the more we can open ourselves to seeing things in a different light. Instead of attaching to this instant, snap judgments, we can *choose* to judge things another way.

As in the example I gave before about feeling bad about not wanting to clean the house, I could release judgment of this thought and consider it with curiosity instead. I could ask myself why I don't want to clean.

Is it because I am tired? Do I have a long to-do list of other things I need to prioritize first? Do I wish that my partner would clean up instead?

If I realize that I am tired and have a busy day ahead, I could do several things to combat this. I could take a nap before diving into my to-do list or make a cup of coffee. I could ask my partner to help. Or I could simply decide to clean later when everything else is finished.

Exploring the thought with curiosity instead of immediately judging has helped me to realize that I am both busy and tired and to realize that I could just ask for help or leave it until later. I also have the added benefit of not wasting additional time on a busy day by getting into a negative thinking spiral.

If you are prone to worrying a lot, the way that I am, it can really help to practice non-judgment. It frees up a lot of time and mental energy that would otherwise simply be spent on worrying.

Benefits of Mindfulness

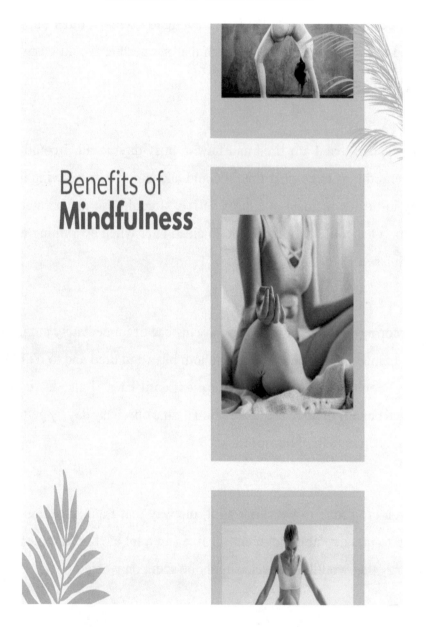

When you practice mindfulness it can benefit your physical and mental health. This includes reducing your general stress level throughout the day.

According to Help Guide,

> **Mindfulness improves physical health.** If greater well-being isn't enough of an incentive, scientists have discovered that mindfulness techniques help improve physical health in a number of ways. Mindfulness can: help relieve stress, treat heart disease, lower blood pressure, reduce chronic pain, improve sleep, and alleviate gastrointestinal difficulties.

> **Mindfulness improves mental health.** In recent years, psychotherapists have turned to mindfulness meditation as an important element in the treatment of a number of problems, including depression, substance abuse, eating disorders, couples' conflicts, anxiety disorders, and obsessive-compulsive disorder.

These numerous benefits of Mindfulness are all great reasons to begin a practice today.

NICOLE DAKE

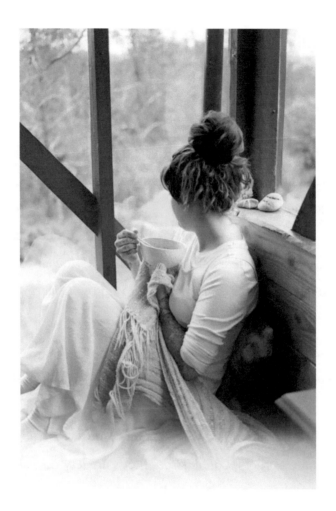

Photo by Callum Shaw on Unsplash

Do you feel like something in your life is off-center? Like you are always just meandering through life, directionless?

Everything is 'fine' on the face of things, but you feel like 'fine' isn't enough to satisfy you. There is something missing.

But what is it? What is that missing piece?

Often, for those of us who are very driven and goal-oriented, the thing that is missing is the enjoyment of the present moment.

This is how I was feeling when I started the Burnout to Badass program and learned how to return to the mindful state that I had been missing for years of my life.

I had heard of mindfulness before when I used to go to meditation classes at a Buddhist temple when I was in my 20s, but it had been years since I had thought about it.

A return to my spirituality through the process of using the mindfulness principle of the Beginners Mind helped me to find peace and clarity and refocus my life in a new direction.

Here are some of the lessons that I learned from Tanvi about mindfulness.

- Mindfulness increases happiness
- Mindfulness helps us be better parents
- Mindfulness helps with Anxiety and Depression
- Mindfulness helps us to fully experience life
- Mindfulness makes us more productive

Now that I have learned how **mindfulness** has improved my life, I want to share this age-old wisdom with all of you here.

Mindfulness increases happiness

When we practice mindfulness, we learn to be present at the moment without judgment.

The non-judgment aspect of mindfulness really helped me learn how to be happier. I have a really harsh inner critic, and by suspending judgment, I no longer had to buy into those self-critical thoughts.

As I was practicing mindfulness, I learned how to let my thoughts just flow past like clouds without attaching to them.

The more we learn to be in the moment, it gets us out of our heads.

We stop constantly analyzing every moment and start living each moment instead.

Mindfulness helps us to fully experience life

Every day, I start the morning by being mindfully present through yoga and sitting on the patio with my coffee. I find that it helps to be outside to begin my mindfulness practice.

Then, just notice everything that is around you. The sights, sounds and smells. The feel of the air on your face. The taste of the coffee. The more you are in the moment, the more able you are to truly see things. The more you begin to really see things around you, the more you can enjoy them.

In order to tap into the present moment, we need to feel it rather than think about it. — Tanvi Chadha

It is through this mindful presence in all the moments of our lives that we learn to be happier and more whole people.

NICOLE DAKE

Mindfulness helps with Anxiety and Depression

Since mindfulness helps us to be more present in our day-to-day experience, to be happier and less judgmental of ourselves, this means it also helps with Anxiety, Depression and other mental health conditions.

Since I was in therapy at the same time I was going through the Burnout to Badass coaching program, I asked my therapist to use the same Buddhist principles in our therapy. I was lucky and blessed to have a therapist who had studied for his master's in counseling at a Buddhist university. So, that made him a great fit for me.

In our sessions, he helped me use mindfulness and loving-kindness meditation to help with my anxiety and depression.

Having allies on your team when you are trying to grow as a person is so valuable. Not only does it help with your mental health, but when multiple professionals explain the same concepts to you in different ways, it helps you understand what to do from different angles.

As I began to practice mindfulness more and more, I learned to cope with not only thoughts that bothered me but with anxious feelings in my body as well. I could look at my symptoms more objectively, and then I could use coping skills more effectively as well.

Mindfulness helps us be better parents

The more mindfully present we are with our children, the better parents we become. We really listen to our kids; we engage with them and play with them instead of being behind our phone screens all the time.

As we become happier, it makes our kids happier too. This is because kids feel and attach to our moods.

Since kids don't understand why people are happy or unhappy, often they will blame themselves when their mom or dad isn't happy.

Therefore, through being more mindful, we can connect better with our kids and help them to have better emotional regulation as well.

NICOLE DAKE

Mindfulness makes us more productive

It may sound counterintuitive since Mindfulness is about slowing down and being present, that mindfulness would also help with productivity, but it does.

People are terrible at multitasking.

The more distracted we are, the longer it takes us to complete any task that we are undertaking. When we are at work, there are often frequent distractions in the form of emails, IMs, calls and texts.

As we become more mindful, we realize that it is OK to turn these distractions off at times so that we can more easily focus on the tasks at hand.

If you work for a company, you can calendar your work time for important tasks the same way you would for a meeting. Then, turn off all your notifications for an hour and see just how much you get done.

Being fully present at the moment helps you with work tasks just as much as it can help you in your personal life.

It can also help you to be more present and engaged, even during boring meetings. The more mindful you are, the more you listen when other people are speaking instead of zoning out or doodling in your notebook.

When you become more present and listen fully and attentively, people notice. Then, your relationships with your colleagues will improve as well.

Mindfulness improves our relationships

I have already discussed how mindfulness can improve your relationships with your children and your colleagues, and it can improve the quality of your romantic relationships as well.

When we take time to be mindful, to fully listen to our partners and be in the moment with them, it helps to deepen our relationships.

Think how often you talk to your partner while watching TV or while one or both of you is on the phone.

As you become more mindful, you learn to put those distractions away. You focus fully on your partner and on the conversation that you are having with them.

This is a way of showing love and respect for our partners and will help to deepen our relationships with them as well.

We get so much of our satisfaction in life from the other people that we spend our lives with. It is important that we be fully present with them so that we can enjoy the best relationships possible.

This goes for friends, family, work colleagues, kids and our partners.

The more mindful we become, the happier we are. This happiness radiates outwards to the people in our lives too.

All these lessons about mindfulness have shown me how bringing this practice into daily life can cause blessings to multiply in so many aspects of your life.

Practicing Mindfulness

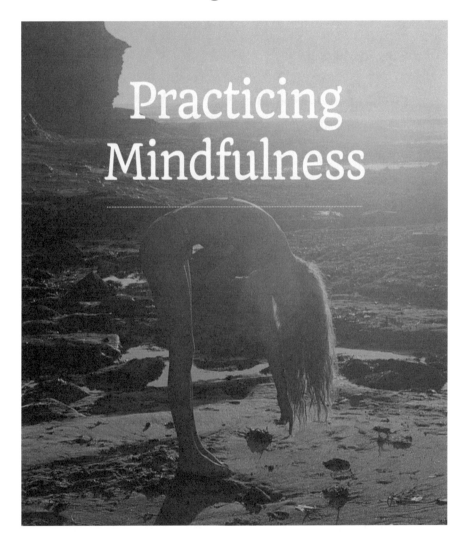

You don't need any equipment to practice mindfulness; all you need is yourself. It is helpful if you first begin your practice in a quiet place.

Personally, I have found that the outdoors or somewhere in nature are good places for me to practice mindfulness.

According to <u>Mindful</u>,

> While mindfulness might seem simple, it's not necessarily all that easy. The real work is to make time every day to just keep doing it. Here's a short practice to get you started:
>
> **Take a seat.** Find a place to sit that feels calm and quiet to you.
>
> **Set a time limit.** If you're just beginning, it can help to choose a short time, such as 5 or 10 minutes.
>
> **Notice your body.** You can sit in a chair with your feet on the floor, you can sit loosely cross-legged, in lotus posture, you can kneel—all are fine. Just make sure you are stable and in a position, you can stay in for a while.
>
> **Feel your breath.** Follow the sensation of your breath as it goes out and as it goes in.
>
> **Notice when your mind has wandered.** Inevitably, your attention will leave the sensations of the breath and wander to other places. When you get around to noticing this—in a few seconds, a minute, five minutes—simply return your attention to the breath.

Be kind to your wandering mind. Don't judge yourself or obsess over the content of the thoughts you find yourself lost in. Just come back.

That's it! That's the practice. You go away, you come back, and you try to do it as kindly as possible.

When you are being mindful, focusing on the breath helps you feel centered within your body.

You can practice mindfulness anywhere, at any time throughout the day. All you have to do is focus on your breath and body and focus on really experiencing the things around you.

To make yourself present in the moment, you can notice the sensations within your body and things within your environment. Notice you're in and out breaths. Notice the wind in the trees and the feel of the air on your skin. Observe if there are sounds in the environment like birds singing.

Being aware of all the sensations within and around you ground you in the present moment.

As I discussed before, the second part of mindfulness is non-judgment.

According to the <u>Harvard Stress Development Lab,</u>

Another key aspect of mindfulness involves acceptance and non-judgment of our present-moment experiences. This includes accepting our thoughts and feelings— whether positive or negative—and immersing ourselves in the present moment without evaluating them.

When your thoughts come, you simply notice them and let them pass without categorizing them as good or bad.

This allows you to create space between yourself and your thoughts.

You are not your thoughts; you are the watcher of your thoughts.

Knowing that your thoughts are separate from yourself; allows you to detach from them. For example, if thoughts are causing you anxiety or stress, knowing that they aren't YOU allows you to release some of your stress.

Once you begin to practice mindfulness, you will start to experience a sensation or quietness, peace and lightness.

Mindfulness has helped me to feel more connected and peaceful in my own life. I hope that it can have the same effect on you!

Beginners Mind is Key to a Growth Mindset

Learn about Beginners Mind in Buddhism and how this can help you constantly grow

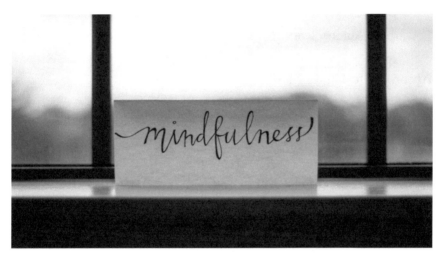

Photo by Lesly Juarez on Unsplash

In the mindset coaching program I took last year in an attempt to find inner peace, I learned about practicing Beginner's Mind. My coach told me to do this exercise in one of my sessions:

Pretend you are an alien. You have never seen anything on earth before. It is all new. Approach everything during the day from this space. What do you appreciate? What questions do you ask yourself? Take nothing for granted.

Growth Mindset

Having a growth mindset means that you think of yourself as constantly learning and evolving. You don't think of things like intelligence or skill as being fixed. You think of them as things that you are constantly learning and improving.

According to Intelligent Change,

> As we mentioned earlier, a growth mindset is an approach to life in which an individual believes that their talents, intelligence, and abilities can be developed further. People with a growth mindset seek opportunities to learn, gain new skills, and enhance their existing skills.

When you have a growth mindset, you realize that you don't know it all. You know that you can constantly improve yourself. It gives you confidence in your ability to learn and grow.

Beginner's Mind and Growth Mindset

When you look at life with a beginner's mind, it helps you to cultivate a growth mindset. You are constantly seeing life and yourself as new and fresh. You are constantly evolving and changing.

PRACTICING BUDDHISM IN EVERYDAY LIFE

You know that you aren't given a fixed skillset at birth that never changes. You can learn new things if you try and apply yourself.

Both a beginner's mind and a growth mindset are about openness.

You are open to yourself, to life, and to an ever-evolving process.

This openness allows you to constantly challenge yourself to learn more. To constantly see new opportunities. To constantly evolve and change, to become better, happier and more full of love.

According to Bodhi,

> Perhaps the most valuable takeaway from studying the Zen Buddhist concept of shoshin was realizing that the beginner's mind is far less limited by false narratives and misconceptions than the fixed mind and, therefore, more open to new possibilities. By shedding our preconceived notions about success and shifting toward a more childlike (process-driven) outlook on life, we may be able to overcome the fear of failure by constantly forcing ourselves to learn and try new things.

Allowing ourselves to be open to new learning lets us move farther in life. It allows us to grow and expand our lives, ourselves, and our skills.

NICOLE DAKE

To be able to grow, we have to learn to see ourselves and the world in a new light. We begin to realize that we don't already know all there is to know. This allows us to be open to new ideas and new ways of doing things.

No matter how advanced we are or how old we are, there is always something new and beautiful to learn about life.

Mindful Parenting: How To Be Present In The Moment With Your Child

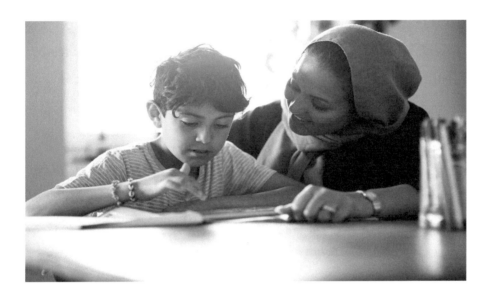

When we parent mindfully, that means that we are present with our kids when we are with them. Being mindful of our kids means paying them our full attention. One of the kids' love languages is Quality Time. That means not just being with someone but having a quality interaction with them.

Put Away Your Phone

I know a lot of moms complain about kids who are constantly on their phones and not paying attention to them. However, it can be just as big of a deal when we are on our phones all the time and not paying close attention to our kids. This can have many negative consequences.

A couple years ago, I had my toddler yell at me, "Mom, put down your phone!" I had been playing an online game instead of playing with her. It really made me realize that this tiny person was feeling like she was in second place to my phone, and she was hurt by it.

According to Very Well Family,

> *When you are with someone, and he is constantly checking, scrolling, texting, or engaged with the cell phone in his hand, it can feel like you are not really fully with that person. "When you have a conversation, it sends a clear message that you are playing second fiddle," says Dr. Roberts. Not only is this behavior rude, but it can damage the quality of that relationship.*

We really do want to make our kids feel loved and prioritized, and it is hurtful to realize that you have been damaging our relationship with our kids. From the point that my daughter yelled at my phone, I make sure to be off my phone when I am spending time with them. If one of them comes to ask me something, I put my phone down and give them my full attention.

In addition to damaging your relationship with your child, being on the phone all the time can also hurt their development. <u>According to the University of Nebraska,</u>

> *Before parents should be concerned about their children's smartphone usage, they should first consider their own. As the ultimate examples of their children, parents need to be mindful of their smartphone consumption since that kind of behavior will set the stage for how children will interact with technology. Parents must consider what image they express to their children and how they communicate responsible smartphone consumption.*

When kids are on smartphones too much as babies and toddlers, it can lead to aggressive behaviors in school, as well as physical health issues. Kids mirror us. When we are on phones too much, they are likely to do the same. Similarly, when we have kids begging us to put the phone down and listen, we really need to be sure we are doing that.

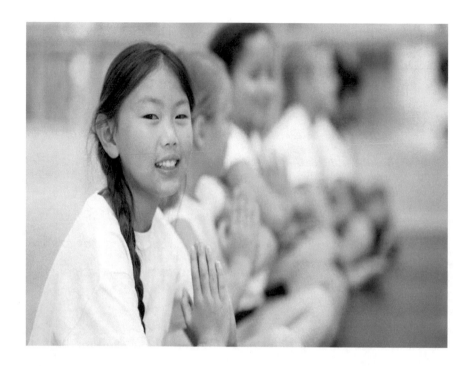

Transformational Listening

Last year I took a class with work that dealt heavily with Transformational Listening, and I learned how much it can truly transform your life when you listen with an open heart. Since I was on work from home when I took the class, I tried practicing all the new listening skills that I learned with my kids. It was really helpful for me to learn to listen to my kids attentively without any devices in front of me.

Even though transformational listening itself is not an aspect of mindfulness, per se, I believe that it has helped me to be mindfully present with my kids, which is incredibly helpful for my relationship with them.

According to Dr. Robin Johnson, "Transformational Listening demonstrates respect behaviorally, helps you collaborate, builds trust, balances extraversion-introversion and direct-indirect communication styles, and is one of the most powerful competencies in the multicultural leader's toolkit.

It is different from active listening since the listener refrains from asking questions or talking while listening to others. The intent of the listener is to connect, demonstrate respect, and learn from the other, while the listener provides the speaker(s) with their undivided caring attention. It is one way of listening to that can be used in addition to (or instead of) active listening."

Dr. Robin has several videos and podcasts available on her website that explain transformational listening in more detail.

I believe the important thing for parents to keep in mind is that listening to our children is important. When we listen with an open heart, it allows our kids to have a feeling of trust and helps them to open up. Although this is important at every age, it can be especially important with teens who often shut their parents out. Building a foundation of trust with our kids from a young age allows them to come to us when they are struggling and to know we will help without judgment.

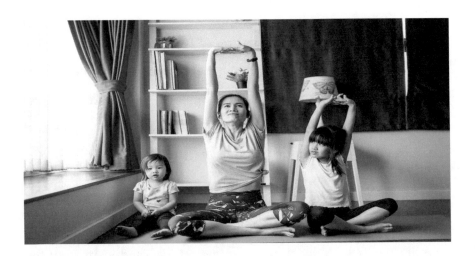

Mindful Parenting

Being a mindful parent is basically the opposite of being a parent who is distracted or uninvolved. It is using your Mindful Presence to be with your kids and be fully immersed in your experience with them. This allows you to make the time that you spend with them into Quality Time.

When you parent mindfully, it allows your children to feel more connected to you. They feel heard, and they feel special. They feel like they are a priority for you because you are willing to put down what you are doing to pay your full attention to them.

According to the <u>Child Mind Institute</u>, the main things that are important for mindful parenting are slowing down and paying attention to your children's needs. This can benefit your children greatly. It also benefits you by creating a calm and less stressed environment in your home.

The Child Mind Institute says that,

> *Your calm response helps kids calm down, too, he notes. "They say, 'Okay, I can trust my parent to be in control; this is a safe environment.' And they feel more secure, and they thrive. So that's another benefit of parents practicing it on their own.*

It seems there's no one right way to parent mindfully. Happily, there are many right ways. Sometimes the smallest adjustment in a child's schedule can change a whole family's day-to-day life. And sometimes, Dr. Bertin says, "It's as simple as practicing paying full attention to our kids, with openness and compassion, and maybe that's enough at any moment.""

There are huge benefits to our children's health and self-esteem when we parent them with mindful attention. Also, it should not be too hard for us to do. Mindfulness can reduce stress. When we parent mindfully and take ourselves away from screens and immerse ourselves in being with our kids, this allows us to be more playful and have more fun too. Children are happy and creative by nature, and taking some of that for us can really help us in addition to them.

Conclusion

Becoming more mindful as parents have many benefits for both our children and us. Mindfulness allows us to focus on the present moment and stop worrying about the past or the future. Being present at the moment allows our kids to feel important and special. It opens the door for them to welcome learning from us.

In addition, we can also learn from our kids through mindfulness. When we are fully immersed in the present moment, we can experience more joy and playfulness, the way that small children already do. Playing with our kids and enjoying the time we spend with them can do so much to enrich our lives through fun.

Mindfulness Quotes to Help You Become a More Peaceful, Happy, and Loving Parent

How mindfulness can help us be more present with our kids in the midst of a busy life.

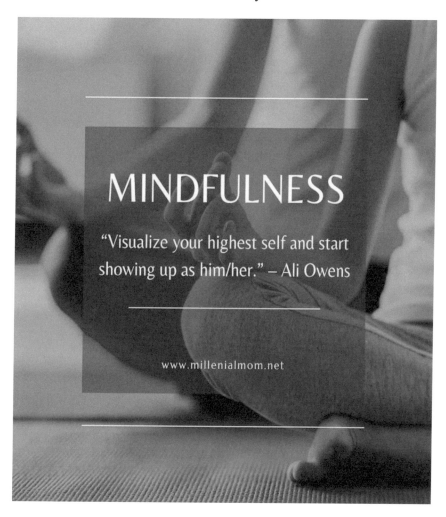

As moms, we have busy, hectic schedules. You probably ask yourself when you will ever get a chance to slow down and get some rest. With little people, those plans often go astray, and we find ourselves making a peanut butter sandwich instead of getting a facial.

Do you feel like things are always moving at such a fast pace that you will never possibly get any time to yourself?

Are you tired and wanting to slow down? To take a breather from all your responsibilities?

If you find yourself having thoughts like this often, it may be time to really slow down and take some time for Mindfulness.

Mindfulness Quotes

"Visualize your highest self and start showing up as him/her."

— Ali Owens

Think about your highest, best self. How does she feel? How does she act? What does she do?

Whatever those qualities you want to have, start acting as if you have them already. If you want to be more brave, do things that scare you. If you want to be more kind, then act with kindness.

You can cultivate more of the qualities that you want to have in your life right where you are already. It just takes practice and conscious awareness. When you act in a mindful way, you will find that you have at least a piece of those qualities within you already.

"Wherever you are, be there totally."
— Eckhart Tolle

This captures the essence of Mindfulness in one line. Be totally immersed in the present moment, no matter where you are or where you are doing.

The more conscious you are of where you are, the less stress you will feel. And, when you feel the stress returning, ask yourself: have you been thinking about the past or the future? That is where stress usually comes from.

There is no stress when we are completely in the moment, simply acceptance. Learn to live mindfully present in the moment, and your stress will begin to melt away.

Having less stress helps us to enjoy our lives more, and be more calm and patient as parents.

> *"Mindfulness gives you time. Time gives you choices. Choices, skillfully made, lead to freedom."*
> — **Bhante Henepola Gunaratana**

Mindfulness allows you to be completely present and aware in each moment of your day. This allows you to consciously decide what you will do in this endless now.

If you just focus on making each moment its best, then you will make better choices. You will be more intentional.

PRACTICING BUDDHISM IN EVERYDAY LIFE

An intentional life is a life of choice and freedom. It is a life where we don't feel like we "have to" do things that we are being forced by outside forces to do. It is a life where we decide what we will do and how we will do it.

When we start from a place of peace and silence, we find better answers than when we are constantly stressed out and in a hurry to go from one thing to the next without appreciating where we are.

> *"Life is a dance. Mindfulness is witnessing that dance."*
> — **Amit Ray**

Life, in all its glory, is beautiful. It is in a constant state of unfolding beautifully and perfectly.

When we really are mindfully present, we allow ourselves to watch life's natural unfolding. As parents, being mindful often means watching our kids and being fully present with them. Kids love to dance. Watch them and learn from them.

Kids are unusually mindful already. Watch the way they notice a beautiful butterfly, a tiny shell, or an odd-shaped rock. They are completely present in their environment and notice things with curiosity.

By paying closer attention to our kids, and to the way they look at things, we become more mindful and peaceful ourselves.

If you ever need some inspiration, just put on some music and let your kids dance. Then, you are seeing the real joy that runs through all life.

"How we pay attention to the present moment largely determines the character of our experience, and therefore, the quality of our lives."
— Sam Harris

When we aren't present in the moment, we aren't enjoying our experience. We are simply doing things half asleep without paying attention to them.

The best day of your life means little if your mind has already jumped ahead to something else. Your mind creates your reality, and the reality is that you create your present moment. You can enjoy it more when you are mindfully present.

Taste every bite of your delicious food. Listen to every cute word that your kids say. Read every page of that book. Being immersed in the activity makes it better; it makes the colors brighter and the smells sweeter.

Conclusion

Once you have learned to be more mindful throughout each day, it helps to enrich your experience of life. Hopefully, these quotes can bring you back to where you are each time your mind strays.

Find one of these quotes that resonate with you and write it down. It can be in your journal or on a note card that you keep with you. Then, you can come back to the quote each time you need to feel more mindful. Eventually, you won't even need to look at it written down; you will remember it well enough to mentally refocus.

The more mindful you are yourself, the better your experience of motherhood will be. You can also set an example of mindfulness for your kids to follow so they don't grow up living stressed-out lives.

To help you teach your kids about mindfulness, here are some Mindfulness for kids activities that you can use during the day.

Being a mindful mom helps you to be less overwhelmed and more focused throughout the day. This can help you to better handle the highs and lows of parenthood.

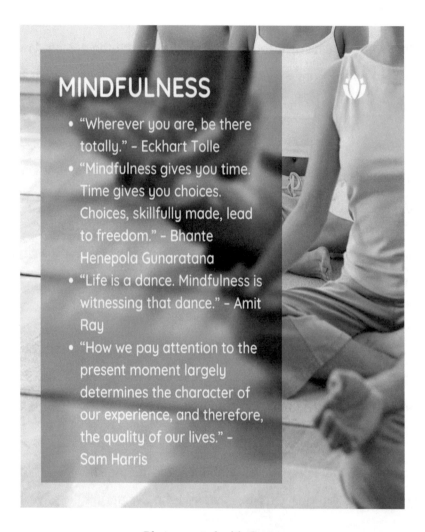

Photo created with Canva

Yoga

My Favorite Way to Relieve Stress Is Doing Yoga

It reduces stress throughout the day.

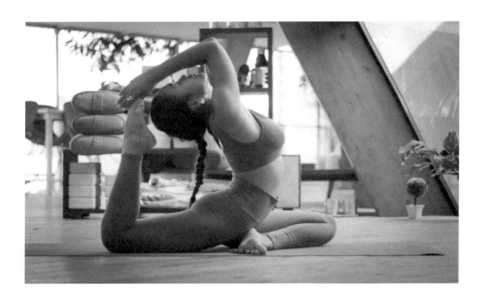

Photo by Carl Barcelo on Unsplash

When I am really stressed, I love to do yoga. I start my day with yoga every day so that I can feel calm and relaxed every morning. That feeling helps to carry with me into the rest of the day.

NICOLE DAKE

I have been doing yoga for about 3 years now, and it has helped me to lower my overall stress levels and to feel more calm and connected to myself.

When I first started doing yoga purely by chance, I was trying to lose weight and started a program called Metabolic Renewal, which starts with a quiz to determine why you are holding onto problem weight.

After taking the quiz, it showed me that I was staying fat because of stress. In addition to the workouts from the program, it advised me to do yoga a couple of times a week to reduce stress.

You heard that right. I was getting fat because of stress.

I didn't stick with Metabolic Renewal, but I am glad that the program helped me discover a yoga practice that I have come to love.

At that point in time, I was going into a crash and burn at a very stressful job that was a bad fit. Ultimately, I ended up quitting the job. But doing yoga helped me create mental space and reduce my stress level for a few minutes each day.

Health Benefits of Yoga

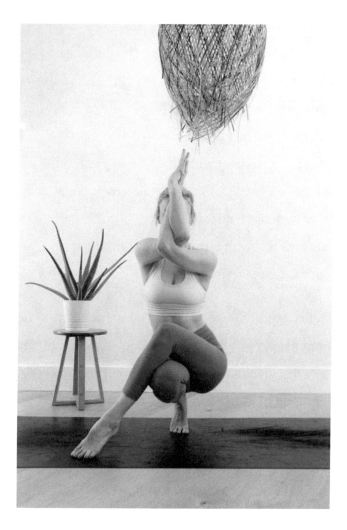

Photo by Sonnie Hiles on Unsplash

There are many benefits to your physical and mental health that come from doing yoga.

According to <u>Johns Hopkins University</u>, some of the benefits of yoga include:

- Improved Strength, balance and flexibility
- Back pain relief
- Eases arthritis symptoms
- Benefits heart health
- Relaxes you to help with sleep
- Contributes to more energy and better moods
- Helps to manage stress
- Connects you with a supportive community
- Leads to better self-care

These benefits can be found even if you are a beginner with yoga and can help people of all ages. You don't have to do the hardest poses to get the greatest benefits. Yoga helps you focus on your breath, be present at the moment, and find mental stillness.

Emotional Benefits of Yoga

Learning yoga has helped me learn to be gentle with myself and to listen to my body. Every day, our body has different needs. Some days, I want fast cardio practice. On other days, I want a slow, gentle stretch. I have learned to accept that it isn't sustainable to push my body to its limits every day. Sometimes, I need to slow down and rest.

PRACTICING BUDDHISM IN EVERYDAY LIFE

There are videos and tutorials for all different styles of yoga and quizzes on what yoga style may benefit you at a given time. Since I mainly started yoga because of stress, I usually try to do a very gentle practice if I am feeling tired or unmotivated.

Yin-style Yoga provides deep, slow stretches to help release tight and sore muscles. It can also help you relax your mind as you focus on your body and your breath.

There is even yoga just for your face to help you release your facial muscles. This can help with reducing stress also.

By teaching us physical balance, yoga also teaches us mental balance. It helps connect our mind to our body through our breathing. There are many balancing poses where you stand on one leg, but that isn't the only aspect of balance. When doing our yoga practice, we keep in balance by repeating each pose for each side of our body. This helps create whole-body balance.

Yoga has also helped me to learn the value of self-acceptance. I think that is something that many of us, as moms, struggle with. We always put our kids and family first (not that it's a bad thing!), but we neglect ourselves in the process. Mom is a part of the family too, and we are deserving of the same care we provide our children.

When we accept ourselves, it is first accepting that we are important and deserve to honor our needs. It is also about accepting where we are in life, with our physical and mental health. We may not be where we want to be in life, but we can still accept that where we are is ok. We can honor our needs in any given moment.

Accepting where we are, accepting ourselves as we are, doesn't mean we give up on our goals. It means that we accept that our goals will take work. And we are still valuable people while we are on the journey to where we want to be. Meeting goals isn't always linear. We can enjoy the process of self-development without putting ourselves down for not being perfect.

Many times when we work on health and fitness goals, it can be easy to bash ourselves for being fat, out of shape, tired, eating chocolate, etc. It is important to do things incrementally and not to be too hard on ourselves. Accept that we are a work in progress. We aren't going to lose 30 pounds by tomorrow in any type of sustainable way.

When I started Yoga, I did 10 minutes a day for months. Then I started doing 15 minutes. Every time I got comfortable with my practice, I would add more time or more difficulty.

But slowly.

Learning to move slowly and gradually really helped me to reduce my stress level overall.

Spiritual Benefits of Yoga

Yoga began as a part of Hinduism and was a practice that was done by the Hindu priest caste. According to Yoga Basics,

> *The beginnings of Yoga were developed by the Indus-Sarasvati civilization in Northern India over 5,000 years ago. The word yoga was first mentioned in the oldest sacred text, the Rig Veda. The Vedas were a collection of texts containing songs, mantras, and rituals to be used by Brahmans, the Vedic priests.*

Since Yoga was originally practiced by priests, it does have a spiritual element to practice. I have experienced this in my own life as I learned to bring my mind and body into alignment through practiced breathing. Focusing on the body and the breath allows my mind to relax. Instead of thinking about what I need to do all day or the past and the future, it allows me to focus on my body and be present.

Being present in my body and feeling my muscles relax into long-held poses in Yin Yoga, I also feel my mind begin to relax. At the end of one yoga practice recently, I was in my Savasana and visualizing light entering my body. I felt this overwhelming feeling of peace, light and love.

It is hard to put into words, but it felt like coming home. It was a feeling of remembrance of our true nature, that of boundless love. We are all a part of one world, one humanity, and we all can have love and compassion for one another. I felt united with that boundless love, and it brought me the true peace that I have been seeking.

The Himalayan Yoga Institute describes it like this,

> *A good yoga practice is one that allows its practitioners to achieve peace — with themselves and the external world they inhabit. The spiritual aspect of yoga emphasizes the attainment of peace and clarity of mind while perfecting the posture is of secondary importance.*

> *When we practice yoga with a spiritual outlook, we acknowledge that the end purpose is transformation and awakening of our true Inner Self. Awakening of Self means realizing our highest potential. Realizing our hidden potential allows us to express the fullness of our divine*

essence and thereby make the greatest possible contribution to the world.

Practicing yoga with this ultimate objective will eventually lead to spiritual fulfillment, a state of great bliss. The practice of yoga aimed at total integration includes a certain lifestyle, the practice of compassion and kindness, and a vegetarian or vegan diet, and all of this plays an important role in the fulfillment of the above objective.

With Yoga, you can make a whole new lifestyle, as they say above. I originally started doing yoga to decrease my anxiety. I believe that it does so on a daily basis. As I have delved more deeply into my yoga practice, I have also returned to a more spiritual and mindful lifestyle.

Yoga doesn't have to be spiritual if you don't choose that for yourself. Although Yoga started with religious people, it is not formally linked to any organized religion today. Yoga itself is not a religion either. You get out of your practice what you choose.

According to <u>Best In Yoga</u>,

> *Yoga is a way to cultivate wholeness. It can help you remember wholeness and recognize it everywhere. For some yogis, wholeness is the spiritual practice of yoga.*
>
> *Spirituality helps you trust in life and yourself, even when managing difficult situations. When you're connected to the self, inner peace grows. You'll find you're more capable of caring and loving for yourself and others, and you'll experience the joy of being who you are by deepening your yoga practice.*

The description of wholeness is what I described as my experience of oneness. First, you come into oneness with yourself. You can align your body, mind and spirit through breath. Then, you may experience a greater oneness as well.

"I am that, you are that, all this is that."

This is an ancient saying about honoring the divine in everyone. It sort of explains the experience of oneness. Here <u>Deepak Chopra</u> addresses it,

To get at the answer [what is that], there's another ancient teaching related to "I Am That," which declares, "This isn't knowledge you learn, it is the knowledge you become." In other words, "That" transforms the person having the experience. Being centered is an everyday experience accessible to anyone. The trick is to let the value of the experience sink in deeply, and then a shift begins. You start shedding the burden of effort and struggle. You begin to see that at its source, silent awareness contains infinite resourcefulness, intelligence, creativity, and love.

Oneness, love and peace are beautiful experiences. I always thought I would have to go to a mountain top somewhere to find it. But to my surprise, it was always waiting here for me to find inside my own house.

Yoga is a great way to counteract the effects of stress. I love yoga because it combines meditation and exercise. When I started my practice, I thought it was the best of both, and I could put in less time by doing one practice for physical and mental wellness.

Getting Started With Yoga

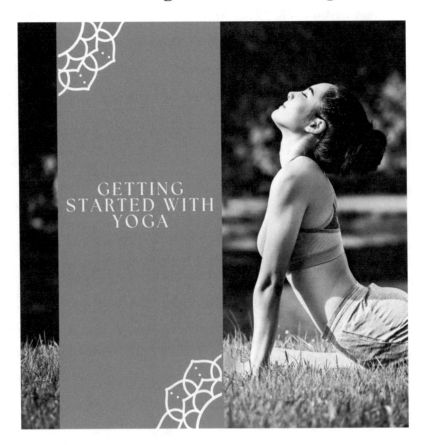

When I started doing yoga, I was a busy mom with a baby that didn't sleep through the night. I was physically and mentally exhausted, and not losing the baby weight. I had heard from some girls that I worked with that yoga was a great easy exercise and even would help with my postpartum anxiety.

I didn't think I had time in my schedule to sign up for an hour-long class at a gym, so I started off with easy videos on YouTube that I could do at home. All I had to buy was a yoga mat!

There are tons of great yoga videos out there and tutorials on how to do different poses. If you follow me on Instagram, I link to them pretty regularly.

This is the first yoga video that I used when I was starting out. I think Sarah Beth does a great job explaining things that are easy to follow. She has a whole playlist with 10-minute, easy beginner videos. That really helped make Yoga accessible to me when I was first starting out.

Another channel that I really love for Yoga is Boho Beautiful. Their videos are sometimes more advanced, but I love all the beautiful locations that they film from.

Yoga with Adrienne is another popular YouTube channel for getting started with a new yoga practice.

When you feel burned out, Yoga is a great way to connect back to yourself. It is wonderful for relaxation, self-care and exercise.

You will get a bunch of wonderful health benefits, as well as the relaxation benefits of meditation.

Different styles of Yoga

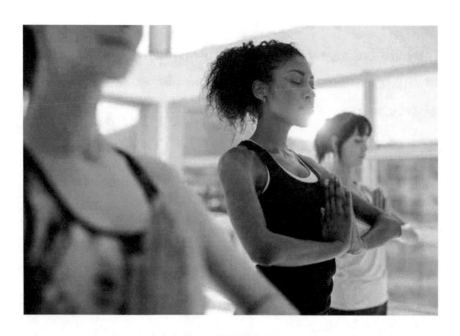

Photo by Wix

There are many different types of yoga out there and choosing which type of yoga is right for you will likely depend on your reasons for wanting to start a yoga practice.

Do you want to do yoga for exercise? Are you interested in reducing anxiety symptoms? Do you want a better balance?

These are just a few of the reasons that women, just like we, have started doing yoga. Here are all the types of yoga and what they can help with! According to <u>Yoga Medicine</u>, here are the different types of yoga.

- **Kundalini Yoga** — This is good for "Anyone in search of a physical, yet also a spiritual practice, or those who like singing or chanting." This type of practice works by "challenging both mind and body with chanting, singing, meditation, and *kriyas (*specific series of poses paired with breath work and chanting). You might notice everyone is wearing white, as it's believed to deflect negativity and increase your aura. Typically, a kundalini class starts with a mantra (a focus for the class), then includes breathing exercises, warmups to get the body moving, increasingly more challenging poses, and a final relaxation and meditation."
- **Vinyasa Yoga** — This is one of the most common styles of yoga that goes through a routine called a flow. "Vinyasa flow is a style of yoga where the poses are synchronized with the breath in a continuous rhythmic flow," says Sherrell Moore-Tucker, RYT 200. "The flow can be meditative in nature, calming the mind and nervous system, even though you're moving." This style of yoga is great for anyone who prefers movement to stillness throughout their yoga practice.

- **Hatha Yoga** — This is a style of yoga focused on creating balance. "The balance in hatha yoga might come from strength and flexibility, physical and mental energy, or breath and the body." Hatha yoga is slower moving, and focused on breath, which makes it a great style for anyone looking for a more gentle type of practice.

- **Ashtanga Yoga** — This style of yoga is great for anyone who likes a routine, which is mostly physical and yet spiritual too. "Ashtanga yoga consists of six series of specific poses taught in order. Each poses and each series is "given" to a student when their teacher decides they have mastered the previous one. This is a very physical, flow-style yoga with spiritual components."

- **Yin Yoga** — This style of yoga is slower, with participants holding their poses for 2 minutes or more. It can be used to stretch out after doing other exercises or by anyone looking for a slower type of practice. Also, "While other forms of yoga focus on the major muscle groups, yin yoga targets the body's connective tissues."

- **Iyengar Yoga** — This type of yoga is good for anyone who wants a more static yoga practice, which is good for any type of physical limitations. "While considered optional in many practices, multiple props are used in Iyengar classes — including chairs, walls, and benches, in addition to more common ones like straps, blocks, and bolsters."

- **Bikram Yoga** — A form of hot yoga, "These classes, like ashtanga classes, consist of a set series of poses performed in the same order, and the practice has strict rules. Each class is 90 minutes, with 26 postures and two breathing exercises, and the room must be 105° Fahrenheit with 40 percent humidity." The purpose of hot yoga is to allow for greater sweat and flexibility.

- **Power Yoga** — Power yoga is a more fast-paced yoga practice with less of a spiritual component. According to practitioners, "power yoga strengthens the muscles while also increasing flexibility. The variation of sequences keeps the brain engaged while you work for all muscle groups in the body."

- **Prenatal Yoga** — Prenatal yoga is a great way for expectant mothers to work out in a gentle way. "Since this is a practice designed specifically for moms-to-be, it excludes poses that might be too taxing or unsafe for the changing body."

Which style of yoga you choose may vary depending on what type of benefits you are looking to get.

You may even choose different styles of yoga on different days once you get a sense of what your body needs. Personally, I tend to alternate between Vinyasa or Power Yoga for exercise, and Yin Yoga for mental clarity and to release stress. Our needs from one day to the next may not be the same, so it is great to try different styles of yoga to meet different needs.

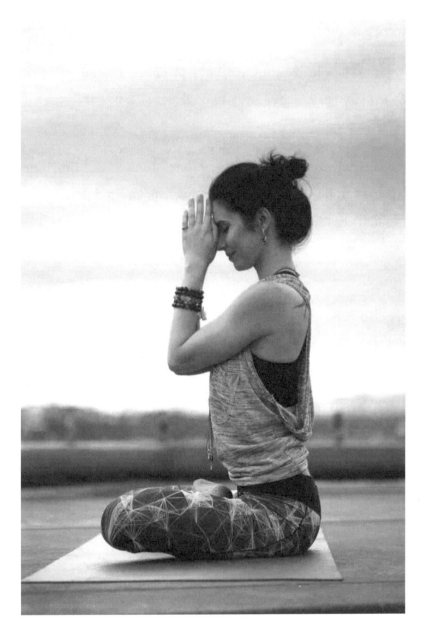

Photo by Wix

Conclusion

Whether you want to improve your physical, mental or spiritual well-being, yoga is a great way to do that!

Since I started doing yoga, I have gained strength and flexibility. I can get up from sitting on the ground with my toddler. I can lift things that are heavier because of the bodyweight exercises. I have toned my arms, legs and abs.

Yoga also helps me to cope with my anxiety better than anything else. I remember when I felt anxious that I could return to my breath. My deep, slow breath at any time can be calming. As yoga calms my mind, I can remember that calm throughout the day by connecting with my breath.

Finally, yoga has helped me feel a return to spirituality. I can connect to a deep peacefulness that I find during yoga at any time that I need it. Once you find peace, you realize that peace is always there.

You can experience these benefits and many others by starting a yoga practice.

Practicing Yoga

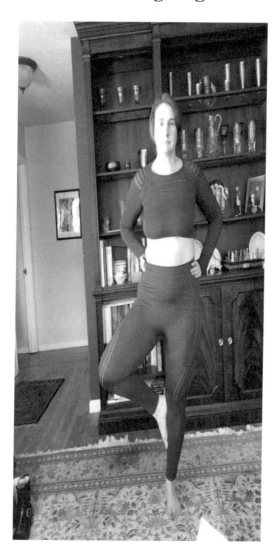

Yoga is called a practice because it acknowledges that we aren't perfect.

NICOLE DAKE

River, my 4-year-old, likes to do yoga with me in the mornings sometimes. The other day our class had us doing a chair pose with a prayer twist, and she said it was too hard.

I told her it was ok and that the teacher had shown a modification of the regular chair pose, and I knew she could do that.

I asked her if she knew why doing yoga was called a practice. She didn't, but you know, she is 4.

I explained that yoga is called a practice because we aren't perfect. We get a little better every day, and eventually, we learn to do harder things.

I told her I couldn't do the hardest version either or take the bind like our teacher. I usually do the medium version of each pose.

She liked that.

Life is a lot like yoga. We can focus on our breath. Relax into things and improve little by little.

I like to teach my kids that we don't have to strive for perfection. Instead, we can focus on getting a little better every day.

That is what I love about yoga. It meets you where you are while helping you become more connected with yourself and more accepting of who you are. As someone who struggles with self-acceptance, this has been important for me.

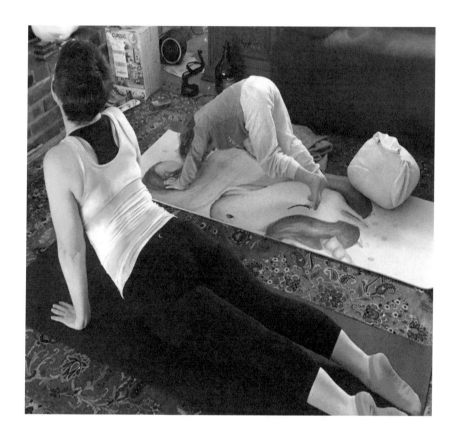

Mom and River Doing Yoga

Meditation

Meditation can help ease stress and calm your mind.

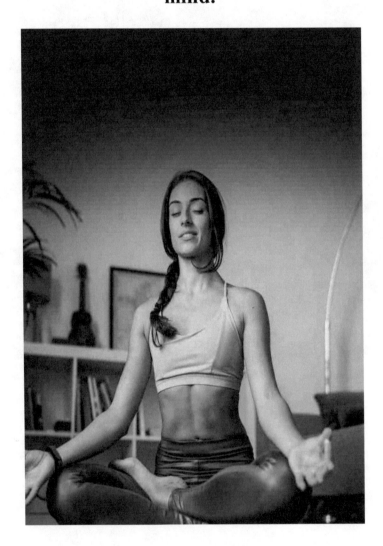

PRACTICING BUDDHISM IN EVERYDAY LIFE

Meditation is a great way to make your mind and your life more peaceful. This is an ancient tradition that is found in many world religions and has also been validated through science as a great way to enrich your life.

According to <u>Very Well Mind</u>, "Research has shown that those who practice meditation regularly begin to experience changes in their response to stress that allow them to recover from stressful situations more easily and experience less stress from the challenges they face in their everyday lives."

There are many other mental and physical health benefits to meditating for even a few minutes a day. You can get started easily using meditation videos on YouTube or meditation music on some of your favorite music apps.

I have meditated on and off for years in many different styles. I find that it makes me calmer, more centered, and more peaceful in my daily life. One of the main things I have learned from meditation is that "You are not your thoughts; you are the watcher of your thoughts." Remembering this idea as I go through daily life is so helpful, especially when I start to think negatively.

When I was in college, I used to go to meditation classes at a Buddhist temple. They had free weekly beginner meditation classes and taught us in detail how to meditate. While I did learn at a Buddhist temple, meditation is not a religious practice. Meditation is about connecting with yourself and learning to calm your mind and body. When you meditate regularly, it can help you feel more relaxed and peaceful in daily life.

A few weeks ago, I started meditating again after several years of substituting yoga for meditation. While yoga is a great way to calm your mind and improve your fitness, meditation has additional benefits.

Meditation and Stress

We all experience stress in many forms throughout our daily lives. However, the effects of chronic stress over time can be very damaging to both our mental and physical health. If we allow stress to overtake us for too long, it can lead to burnout, depression, anxiety, heart problems, and a host of other issues.

The Centre for Studies on Human Stress defines chronic stress as "…stress resulting from repeated exposure to situations that lead to the release of stress hormones." They caution that "This type of stress can cause wear and tear on your mind and body. Many scientists think that our stress response system was not designed to be constantly activated. This overuse may contribute to the breakdown of many bodily systems." (BetterHelp)

Some of the effects of chronic stress on your body, according to BetterHelp, can include:

- High blood pressure
- Heart disease
- Elevated heart rate
- Diabetes
- Getting sick often due to suppression of the immune system
- Ulcers
- Erectile dysfunction
- Fertility problems
- Low sex drive
- Irregular menstrual periods
- A decrease in muscle tone
- Insomnia
- Headaches

Meditation is a great way to reduce stress in your life because it helps you to calm your mind and lower your stress response. Meditation is one of many good health behaviors you can use to reduce chronic stress over time in your own life.

This can include stress from work, your finances, relationships, kids, or anything else that is making you constantly feel like you are under stress.

According to Very Well Mind,

> *Meditation affects the body in exactly the opposite way that stress does — by triggering the body's relaxation response. It restores the body to a calm state, helping the body repair itself and preventing new damage from the physical effects of stress. It can calm your mind and body by quieting the stress-induced thoughts that keep your body's stress response triggered.*

Since I have recently started to meditate again, I find myself less triggered by daily events that seem like a nuisance. Instead of becoming upset and stuck in negative emotions about problems with kids or work, I skip blaming and getting upset instead of going right to problem-solving.

When you have kids, there are tons of things that happen daily that can be stressful. My toddler resists her bedtime. My teens leave a bunch of take-out containers smelling up the refrigerator. My partner gets irritated with what the kids are doing. Small things, but when you have these situations being hurled at you all day long and have the family relying on you to fix not only their problems but their emotions about the problems, it can become very taxing and stressful for everyone.

Meditation helps me find a calmer mind so that it takes longer for me to get stressed out about day-to-day things that happen. It is then easier for me to deal with life's problems without having to deal with my own upset feelings in addition.

In therapy, I have learned to look at stress as a continuum. My therapist has me rate my stress level on a scale from 1–10, where 1 is no stress, and 10 is so overwhelming it is going to cause a panic attack.

When we are carrying around a load of stressors all the time, our baseline level of stress, or the way we feel all the time, is higher. If I am under a lot of stress all the time, my baseline might be around a 7 or 8, without anything needing to "happen" to be causing that stress level. But when I meditate, it can lower that baseline level of stress so that I can more easily handle my stress without it leading to a panic attack.

Most people don't have panic attacks, but you may instead have an unwanted outburst and end up yelling at your kids or your partner more easily over situations that come up throughout the day. Meditation can calm your nervous system and help you stop being that yelling, mom.

Other Benefits of Meditation

In addition to reducing stress, there are many other benefits to your physical and mental health. These, in turn, can benefit your relationship with your kids and your partner and help you to be more calm and healthy in your day-to-day life.

According to Healthline, some of the other benefits of meditation are that it:

- Controls Anxiety
- Promotes Emotional Health
- Enhances Self-Awareness
- Lengthens Attention Span
- May reduce age-related memory loss
- Can generate kindness
- May help fight addictions
- Improves sleep
- Helps control pain
- Can decrease blood pressure
- Accessible anywhere

All of these benefits can help you be a happier, more focused and calmer mom. I find myself being more patient as I practice meditation, and things upset me less often with my kids. So, meditation makes me a better mom. When we are happier and healthier, our kids can be happier and healthier too.

How to Meditate?

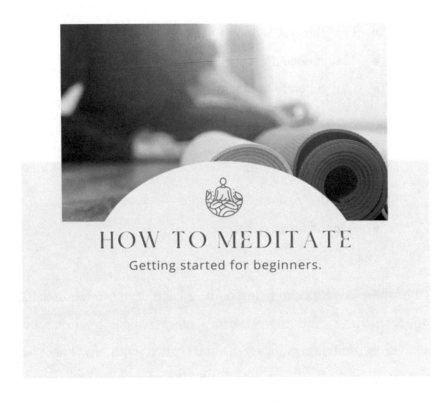

HOW TO MEDITATE
Getting started for beginners.

There are many different types of meditation, which can be found through Buddhist or secular teachings. You can go to a meditation class, or you can meditate anywhere. All you have to do is close your eyes and focus inward on your breath.

It can help to create a calm and relaxing space before you meditate. You can set aside a certain space in your house and light candles or find a quiet place outdoors. Anything that helps you to feel calm is great.

Typically, I will listen to a meditation tape right before I go to bed so that I can feel peaceful and relaxed for sleep, but you can also start your day with meditation. Or, if you want, you can meditate anytime throughout the day when you are feeling stressed. You can take a break at your desk or go for a walking meditation outside.

Here are some tips on getting started with meditation, step by step, from Mindful.

Meditation is simpler (and harder) than most people think. Read these steps, make sure you're somewhere where you can relax into this process, set a timer, and give it a shot:

1) **Take a seat:** Find place to sit that feels calm and quiet to you.

2) **Set a time limit:** If you're just beginning, it can help to choose a short time, such as five or 10 minutes.

3) Notice your body: You can sit in a chair with your feet on the floor, you can sit loosely cross-legged, and you can kneel — all are fine. Just make sure you are stable and in a position, you can stay in for a while.

4) Feel your breath: Follow the sensation of your breath as it goes in and as it goes out.

5) Notice when your mind has wandered: Inevitably, your attention will leave the breath and wander to other places. When you get around to noticing that your mind has wandered — in a few seconds, a minute, five minutes — simply return your attention to the breath.

6) Be kind to your wandering mind: Don't judge yourself or obsess over the content of the thoughts you find yourself lost in. Just come back.

7) Close with kindness: When you're ready, gently lift your gaze (if your eyes are closed, open them). Take a moment and notice any sounds in the environment. Notice how your body feels right now. Notice your thoughts and emotions.

That's it! That's the practice. You focus your attention, your mind wanders, you bring it back, and you try to do it as kindly as possible (as many times as you need to)."

You can play meditation music in the background, chant "Om" to yourself, or choose to sit quietly. If you would like an example of how to meditate, there are some great guided meditations on YouTube.

The purpose of meditation is to find calm and peace, and it can greatly enrich your life if you add it to your daily routine. Remember, be gentle with yourself as you are starting. It is easy to get distracted when you are first starting out, and that is why I recommend guided mediation if you are a beginner. Then, once you get used to it, you can easily meditate anytime you feel like you need it.

Chant the "Om" and Remember How to Fly

When you go into meditation, you become one with your highest self again.

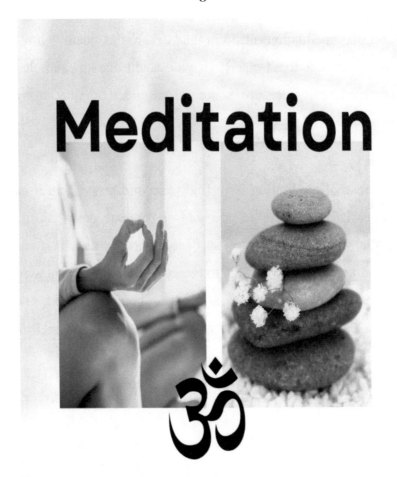

Chant the "OM" and remember how to fly.

Photo created with Canva

When you aren't at one with yourself, you have a tendency to struggle through life. This is true for each one of us.

We may have forgotten to do our daily yoga or meditation practice or have been faced with a challenging circumstance and become caught up in it.

Don't beat yourself up when this happens.

Easier said than done, I know. But beating yourself up doesn't help. It just takes you farther into a dark spiral and farther away from your true nature.

Our true nature is one of pure, perfect peace. It is an inner space of love, light and wholeness. We can tap into that quiet space inside in many ways.

Why Om?

The Om syllable is used as a sacred chant within Hinduism and Buddhism. You may just chant Om all by itself, or you may chant an Om mantra.

According to MBG Mindfulness,

> *Om is a foundation of Hinduism, where it is considered*

the very first sound of the universe. "Before the sound Om, there was nothing," Vasavi Kumar, LMSW, MSEd, a RYT-200 ashtanga yoga teacher, tells mbg.

When said aloud, Om (or Aum) actually sounds like a three-part word. "The A represents creation, U is a manifestation, and M is destruction," explains Kumar. "It's basically all-encompassing—the whole universe joined into a single sound. It represents the union of the mind, body, and spirit."

Deepha Sundaram, Ph.D., assistant professor of religious studies at the University of Denver, adds, "The Om symbol represents unification within Hinduism. People think about Om as a way to bring those three parts of your self—the mind, the body and the spirit—together."

Om also has ties to Buddhism, where it refers to compassion and connection. And in Jainism, it's often used in reference to Pañca-Parameṣṭhi, or the five supreme beings of the ancient Indian religion.

If you close your eyes and meditate to an Om chant, it can help you start to feel centered within yourself and within the world again.

Chant the Om. Breathe. Repeat.

Focus only on the syllable and on your breath. Feel your chest moving up and down. Feel the air on your skin.

In breath. Out breath. Om. Repeat.

Om Mantras

Personally, when I meditate, I usually use a recording of the **Om Mani Padme** Hum chant. This is also known as the mantra of ultimate compassion within Buddhism.

According to YogaPedia,

> Om Mani Padme Hum is a well-loved Buddhist mantra commonly translated as, "The jewel is in the lotus."

This may seem like a strange thing to chant. However, there is a deeper meaning behind each syllable of this mantra.

YogaPedia Continues,

> **This is to say that within all of us is the lotus flower; it's just covered up by a lot of mud and muck.**
>
> Reciting this mantra over and over again, with the right intention, is believed to get rid of the mud and muck until we are as sparkling, pure, compassionate and wise

NICOLE DAKE

as the lotus flower itself.

Via Youtube

Some other Om mantras that are frequently chanted are Om Namah Shivaya and Om Gum Ganapatayei Namah. You can find more mantras that you can use on <u>Meditative Mind</u> if you are interested in learning more about other mantras.

In addition to YouTube videos that you can use to listen to Om chants, they are also available on Apple Music and other music apps. You can also download meditation-specific apps.

Whatever you choose, from my heart to yours, I wish you peace.

The Search to Reclaim Inner Peace

Take time to unwind at the end of the day

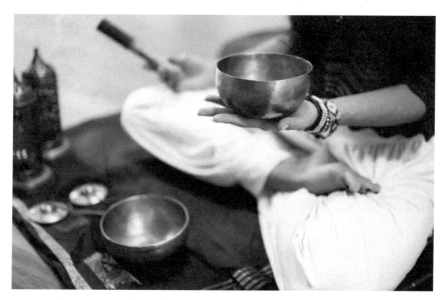

Photo by <u>Conscious Design</u> on <u>Unsplash</u>

- Do you start the day with meditation, yoga or mindfulness, but then find that your day steals the peace that you find there?

- Do you let the worries of the day consume you and fall into bed feeling exhausted?

- Do you want to find a way to get back that feeling of peace from the morning and go to bed feeling peaceful too?

It isn't as impossible as it may seem at times.

Self-Care time

If you are anything like me, you probably thrive on your morning routine and start the day off with a bang.

Everyone in self-help (myself included) stresses the important of a morning routine to set the tone for the rest of the day. Whether you take a cold shower, journal, go for a run, or do yoga in the morning, you are putting yourself first at the beginning of the day.

The problem is, the rest of the day happens. Sometimes things happen that we have no control over, and we let them steal our peace.

Recently I was reading "How to Live Your Best Life" by Maria Hatzistefanis (highly recommend), and she talks about having a routine for the end of the day too. This way, you can separate from the stressors of the day and do something good for yourself.

You don't have to end the day as a couch potato watching forgettable shows on Netflix while mindlessly scrolling through your phone.

So, when you get out of work or after dinner, take some more time to do something good for yourself.

You can do a short meditation, listen to some relaxing music, take a hot bath with some candles lit and unwind.

Or, you can take a page out of Maria's playbook and go out and do something self-indulgent. Go grab a coffee and listen to some jazz, go shopping, try out a new café or go to an art gallery.

Whether you decide to opt for self-care or self-indulgence in the evenings, doing something good for your own well-being and piece of mind will help you to have something to look forward to all day. The mornings won't be your only time to shine anymore.

Closing Thoughts

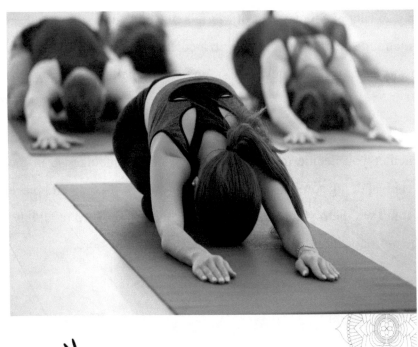

Mindfulness, yoga and meditation are great ways to bring Buddhism into your everyday life. With these practices, you can achieve amazing physical and mental health benefits, relieve stress, and find inner peace and spiritual realization.

The more you practice Buddhism, the more you become in tune with yourself.

As you begin to deepen your practices, you will become more and more of yourself. And as you practice throughout your lifetime, you can find more and more of the peace and love that is the essence of your innermost being. The inner being of all that is, all that was, and all that will be. You are a part of the Prana, the life force that runs through everything that lives.

When you begin to open your mind to open your heart, through using these scientifically validated Buddhist practices, you will come to find more of your truest self.

I hope that you will be able to find this peace and love within yourself more and more each day. As you do so, I hope that it enriches your life beyond measure the way it has mine.

References

- https://wewearwellness.com/work-with-me/
- Sadguru, Shadguru: 11 definitions (wisdomlib.org)
- The Four Noble Truths: Essence of the Dhamma | Buddho.org
- https://www.youtube.com/channel/UC-0CzRZeML8zw4pFTVDq65Q
- Living Buddha, Living Christ by Thich Nhat Hanh: 9781594482397 | PenguinRandomHouse.com: Books
- Meditation and Mindfulness: What You Need To Know | NCCIH (nih.gov)
- Harvard researchers study how mindfulness may change the brain in depressed patients – Harvard Gazette
- The research-backed benefits of yoga (medicalnewstoday.com)
- What Is Mindfulness? - Headspace
- Seven Essential Attitudes of Mindfulness – Mindful Adventure
- Approaching Life with Beginner's Mind - zen habits zen habits
- Non-Judgment: What is it? And Why Does it Matter? (4 Benefits) | Mindful Ambition
- Benefits of Mindfulness - HelpGuide.org
- How to Practice Mindfulness - Mindful
- Mindfulness - Acceptance and Non-Judgment | Stress & Development Lab (harvard.edu)
- What Is Growth Mindset and How to Achieve It – Intelligent Change
- Shoshin: Having a "Beginner's Mind" Can Improve Your Life • Bodhi Surf + Yoga
- Can Too Much Cell Phone Usage Hurt Your Family Bond?

(verywellfamily.com)
- The Effect of Smartphones on Child Development | CUNE Online
- Listening | Robin Denise Johnson, Ph.D. (drrobinjohnson.com)
- Practice Mindful Parenting | Mindfulness Techniques | Child Mind Institute
- Teach Kids to Stop and Smell the Roses with These Mindfulness Activities - Simply Rooted Family
- 9 Benefits of Yoga | Johns Hopkins Medicine
- History of Yoga • Yoga Basics
- The Spiritual Side of Yoga – What it Means and How to Achieve it – Himalayan Yoga Institute
- https://bestinyoga.com/spiritual-benefits-of-yoga/
- "I Am That": A Secret Teaching Comes Home for All of Us (chopra.com)
- Types of Yoga: A Guide to the Different Styles - Yoga Medicine
- The Benefits of Meditation (verywellmind.com) The Benefits of Meditation (verywellmind.com)
- Acute vs. chronic stress - CESH / CSHS (humanstress.ca)
- Chronic Stress: How It Affects You And How To Get Relief | BetterHelp
- The Benefits of Meditation (verywellmind.com)
- Are you coping with PTSD and panic attacks as a busy mom? (millenialmom.net)
- Benefits of Meditation: 12 Science-Based Benefits of Meditation (healthline.com)
- How to Meditate - Mindful
- What Does The Om Symbol Mean? History & How To Use It | mindbodygreen
- The Meaning of Om Mani Padme Hum (yogapedia.com)

- <u>10 Powerful Mantras That Will Transform Your Life |</u>
<u>MeditativeMind</u>

About the Author

Nicole Dake is a blogger, author, and mom of two. Nicole blogs about parenting, mental health, and spirituality. Nicole has a BA in Psychology with a minor in Religious Studies from the University of Colorado and Paralegal Certification from Boston University. Currently located in Beverungen, Germany. Originally from the US.

Nicole is also a Spiritual Life Coach and ordained minister of the Universal Life Church Monastery.

Published works: *Trauma Survivor's Guide to Coping with Panic Attacks* **(2021),** *Happy. Healthy. Rich. The smart mom's guide to living your best life.* **(2021***) and The Way Things Go, A book of poems* **(2022),** *Daily Positive Affirmations* **(2022),** and *A Narcissist Destroyed my Life: How do I Rebuild?* **(2022***).*

Made in the USA
Columbia, SC
15 January 2024

30479012R00078